# Women, Violence and Social Stigma

# Women, Violence and Social Stigma

## A Sociology of Burn Attacks

L. Allen Furr

RAWAT PUBLICATIONS
Jaipur • New Delhi • Bangalore • Guwahati • Kolkata

ISBN 978-81-316-0935-4



*Published by*
Prem Rawat for **Rawat Publications**
Satyam Apts, Sector 3, Jawahar Nagar, Jaipur 302 004 (India)
Phone: 0141 265 1748 / 7006 Fax: 0141 265 1748
E-mail: info@rawatbooks.com
Website: www.rawatbooks.com

*New Delhi Office*
4858/24, Ansari Road, Daryaganj, New Delhi 110 002
Phone: 011 2326 3290

Also at *Bangalore, Guwahati* and *Kolkata*

Typeset by Rawat Computers, Jaipur
Printed at Chaman Enterprises, New Delhi

*To the memory of my sister Patsy White*

# Contents

# Acknowledgements

Every work such as this is produced not just by an author, but also by a number of folks who provide support and insight that made the book possible. All too infrequently they do not know how important they are to an author. If there is anything good in this book, it is because of their contributions, support, encouragement, and feedback. Whatever may be wrong is my responsibility. I am thankful to a number of good people who helped me find my way in writing this book, and I am in their debt.

First, this book was very much a family affair. My wife, Abby Shapiro, allowed me many absences from home to travel to India and immerse myself in the society and culture often for extended periods of time. Not only did she tolerate and encourage my journeys to collect data, teach, and generally become more culturally acculturated, but she also read earlier versions of this manuscript with a sharp critical eye, solving many problems that I found myself in. My daughter, Anna Furr, also endured my trips to India and helped develop this manuscript, and my niece, Margaret Payne, provided expert criticism and editorial assistance.

Many friends and colleagues played important roles in putting this work together. I want to extend special gratitude to John Barker, who some 16 years ago introduced me to the problems surrounding severe facial disfigurement. His wisdom, expertise, and resolve to comfort those in distress have influenced me in immeasurable ways. Keeping up with John's fountain of ideas and willingness to dive into uncharted research waters has tested my own wits on numerous occasions.

I also want to thank my friend Harvinder Bhatti of Punjabi University in Patiala. We first met in 2005, when I was a Fulbright Scholar, because of a last-minute change in assignment that redirected me to Patiala from another destination – it was the greatest stroke of luck. We have maintained our collaborations and friendship well into our second decade now, and he and his family have made Patiala my home away from home.

I appreciate the help of Geetha Suresh and A. Srikrishnan who assisted with the original data collection and translations, and Cynthia Negrey of the University of Louisville for helping me work through the initial ideas of this project. Janice Clifford of Auburn University provided valuable comments on a draft of the original paper on stigma, and Kristrina Shuler, also of Auburn, proffered keen insights on the anthropology of the body. I also want to thank the University of Louisville for funding the original data collection.

Thanks also go to Claire Renzetti, the editor of *Violence Against Women*, for granting consent to reproduce parts of my study, 'Facial Disfigurement Stigma: A Study of Victims of Domestic Assaults with Fire in India', which was published in that journal in 2014.

Last, and certainly not least, I want to express my sincerest appreciation to Rawat Publications in Jaipur. The editors and staff have shown interest and support for this project since the beginning, and I am most grateful.

# Preface

I remember this particular summer in southern India and its hot, humid, stifling air. It wasn't my first trip to India; it wasn't even my first summer there. But I remember the air that day, the aromas it carried and the emotions it portended.

My two associates and I climbed the dark, dingy steps to the third floor of an apartment building nestled tightly in a low-income neighborhood in the heart of the city. I was there to meet and interview a young woman whose husband, I was told, had doused her with kerosene and then threw a lighted match on her, sending her clothes and skin into blistering, searing flames. Our meeting was secret; if her husband or his relatives learned she had spoken to me, she would have hell to pay. We were conducted up the stairs by a female relative of the woman I was there to meet. Our guide, a quiet woman in her 40s, looked over her shoulder a few times to ensure we were not detected. Thc prccautions taken to prevent the victim's husband or his family from knowing about the interview appeared successful. We were alone.

I felt damp as we ascended the narrow steps. Never one to shun such excitement, I felt adrenalin surge through my veins as I collected my thoughts on how I would approach the woman and engage her in conversation. I was not a stranger to experiences somewhat out of the ordinary. I was excited and ready to go.

We reached the top of the stairs and were led to the back room of the small flat. There was only dim, natural lighting, and a few pieces of furniture filled the space between the concrete walls. The air was heavy, but surprisingly not as hot as I thought it would be, the shade and the dampness made the room relatively cool compared to outside. The air was a bit stuffy, but not uncomfortably so.

We walked through the flat to the back room where two other women were introduced to me as her relatives and who appeared to be in their 50s and were draped in colorful saris. They had serious, but accepting expressions on their faces. They likely had never met an American or a professor before and met me with a dignified deference and respect. With the advantages of hindsight, I still cannot say why they agreed to meet me and allowed me to talk to their disfigured and endangered relative. They knew I was not a physician and that I was only interested in hearing their stories. After introductions, I was directed to the person I was there to see.

Lying on a small bed with her face partially covered was 'Gita'. Her hair was pulled back and braided in a South Indian fashion, and she wore a beautiful, dark blue sari. There was little light on her, but I could see she had strong features. Although she lay prone and motionless, she seemed tall, even athletic in appearance. As I sat down and thanked her for meeting with me, my demeanor and sense of purpose changed as if on a switch. Almost immediately I knew this 'case' was not going to be included in my study.

Gita began to tell her story of her deeply troubled marriage and the violence she experienced almost daily. In a startling display given the modesty standards in India, she showed me her wounds. Hand-sized bruises, fresh blood still in the skin. Small burns from cigarettes dotted her arms. And then she bared her upper shoulders, neck, and full face to reveal the scars that betrayed the worst day of her life – the day her husband doused her with kerosene and set her ablaze. Fortunately for her, other people were close by and responded to her screams and extinguished the fire before the fire could spread to her lower body. Somehow her hair was only singed. And that made her 'lucky'.

Having worked on a face transplantation research team for several years, I was accustomed to seeing disfigurement such as hers and worse. What I was not prepared for, however, was the context and the danger in which she lived. She still resided with the husband who had beaten her the night before we met, as evidenced by the fresh contusions and burns, and lived in constant fear of the next assault that would certainly come to her. Her main worry was that the violence would eventually be directed towards her two young children. She felt hopeless, afraid, and trapped.

'Gita' is not included in this research on the stigma associated with facial disfigurement. Her face was largely spared by the flames that could have easily taken her life. Plus, and more importantly, participating in the study could have placed her in additional danger. Nonetheless, she had more influence on me than any person I met during the duration of this study. She was among the first disfigured women I met in India, and though I would soon meet a number of other women who were more seriously scarred than she, none would have the emotional impact of teaching me the horror of an intimate partner attempting to burn them to death.

Though probably not her intent, she became the representation of the status of women in my mind. Now I had a face to associate with the statistics that a fourth to a third of all women in India are subject to intimate partner violence and that 2 per cent of all women in India, which is roughly 9 to 10 million women, have been burned in various degrees by their partners. The problem I was studying was not inconsequential.

Our conversation lasted about 30 minutes, and we left as secretly as we had arrived. We drove away safely amidst the noise and congestion of a large metropolis to our next appointment. She walked to her home and returned to her nightmare.

Despite my experience in India and working with facial disfigurement, meeting Gita was, and still is, my most sobering professional moment. I had been a part of a research team pioneering face transplantation, writing papers on ethics of the surgery and the psychosocial quality of life of severely disfigured persons. We were involved with people whose faces had burned away – noses, ears, eyelids, lips, and skin destroyed by the ravages of fire stemming from an auto crash. Others had their faces destroyed by cancer or trauma from occupational or other accidents. We were looking for an alternative to the usual processes of facial reconstruction, which involves scores of surgeries, considerable expense, and results that often fail to restore patients to a 'passable' appearance. In other words, reconstruction for severely disfigured persons rarely returns them to any sense of physical normalcy.

As a consequence, disfigured persons often live lives of isolation as they avoid uncomfortable stares, inappropriate questions, and insulting comments. They are rejected frequently by others because their appearance is off-putting, even frightening to some. Our hope was that face transplantation had a better chance of restoring an acceptable appearance and allowing these unfortunate individuals to return to an engaging and satisfying social life. Francis Macgregor (1951, 1990), the psychologist who largely initiated the study of the effects of disfigurement on psychological and social well-being, described severely disfigured people metaphorically as 'socially dead'. Confronting the prejudice and discrimination that others display, disfigured people isolate themselves, hiding in their homes that provide the social distance that makes them safe from the torment of others. For many disfigured individuals, social avoidance becomes a central psychosocial theme; while it may offer protection from punishing interactions with others, it often causes them to retreat from themselves as well, leading to depression and an increased risk of suicide.

In time, our transplantation research ended, and our team members scattered to other professional endeavors. I had made several trips to India and Nepal for other research and teaching projects, and during those years, media reports of incidences in which men were setting women on fire with kerosene or throwing acid on women's faces proliferated. Scholars and physicians, primarily in South Asia, were also looking into the problem and produced a fairly large number of research articles on the rates of burn assaults, the causes of the attacks, and the treatment of burns. Researchers, however, only studied the period of time that included the lead-up to the attack, the attack itself, and the immediate days and weeks afterwards in which medical treatment was rendered. No one seemed to be interested in these women five to ten years following the tragic event. The study reported here seeks to remedy that dearth in knowledge.

This book seeks to make sociological sense of the stories of Indian women who have been set afire by husbands in the course of some domestic problem. As mentioned above, the attacks and their immediate consequences have been well documented in numerous testimonials and media accounts. What is missing, however, is the story of the years following the attacks and how victims are never freed from the stigma of being disfigured. One man renders them scarred; society treats them as perpetual outcasts. How does this happen? These are women who otherwise are perfectly healthy and functional, yet because their appearance is marred by fire, they are seen as having little worth or appeal and are often shunned by their closest relatives.

After women are attacked with fire, they experience two more traumas in their lives. First, society changes their identities from who they were before the attack to a new identity that includes being disfigured. They are no longer 'a woman'; they are transformed into 'a burned woman'. Second, because that identity change is dramatic and permanent, disfigured women are treated differently from other women. Believed to be tainted and defective, disfigured women to varying degrees are socially excommunicated. Some friends and relatives abandon them; others fear them. Strangers ridicule and exploit them. Few disfigured women in India have an easy life, their chances for employment are poor and for a stable marriage, even lower. Depression is routine, suicide attempts are common, and feelings of being lost and alone are everyday companions.

Although the book is about the lives of disfigured women after they were burned, it is necessary to try to understand the context in which they were attacked in this manner. To understand the stigma attached to disfigurement, we must first know something about being a woman in India. Therefore, we will spend some looking at the social context of gender in the country and why and how women are burned intentionally. The argument presented here follows a logic train of several theoretical propositions.

*Proposition 1:* The female body is essentialized or reduced down to a small social role by a patriarchal ideology.

*Proposition 2:* This social location means that women are of low value and can be discarded by fire, an act of purification, when deemed necessary.

*Proposition 3:* Those who survive the fire that was accelerated with kerosene are left with a scarred and disfigured body, which causes them to enter a new social status – that of a burned woman.

*Proposition 4:* This new status is stigmatized, even demonized by others, causing hardships and a struggle to enjoy to life.

It is my hope that the pages that follow will help readers to better understand the stigma and discrimination that disfigured women face in India.

Chapter 1 begins the analysis by outlining the major themes in the study. Here I discuss the ideas that serve as axioms guiding the study: the significance of the human face and the meaning and consequences of disfigurement; a brief discussion of fire in the Indian cultural context; and the position of women in Indian society. One of the themes of the book is that the social and cultural realities of gender result from different social interpretations of the body. Female and male bodies are different entities in this way of thinking, resulting in a split within the human population that in turn implies different expectations of behavior, attitudes, and social position. When the body, particularly the face, is disfigured, the body becomes yet another 'thing', and the rules of interpreting it change along with appearance.

Chapter 2 explores the social position of women and the significance of female appearance in some depth in order to provide a context for the direction that disfigurement stigma takes. The experiences of disfigured Indian men will not be discussed here, because the extent literature on burn assaults indicates a gendered patterns of victim and victimizer. Disfigurement stigma in India appears to follow suit and is a gendered phenomenon as well. I argue that women are essentialized, which means that women are reduced to a basic set of expectations that are not equal to those of men. Women are experienced by men (as well as some women) as an 'other' and are interchangeable, which means that a woman can be easily replaced with another. I've converted 'essentialized' to a verb that represents the process by which women are intentionally burned and then discriminated against because of their subsequent scars and wounds. This chapter attempts to argue that women with disfigurement experience is largely a function of a top-down social and ideological conception of women as existing to serve the needs and aspirations of men.

Chapter 3 reviews the literature on burn assaults. Incidence and prevalence are discussed, as are attempts to explain the violence. Using survey data from the Demographic and Health Surveys (DHS), Chapter 3 also attempts to create a profile of women who survived severe burns by their husbands. The DHS is an excellent data source on women's general health and well-being. In recent years, DHS, which conducts similar data collections across the globe, has asked about domestic and intimate partner violence, clearly defining violence as a public and women's health issue. The sample is randomly selected, no small achievement at the national level in India, which allows us to generalize to the population and make rough estimates of that population's overall characteristics. Chapter 3 also discusses treatment options for severe disfigurement to show that medical remedies are not able to reverse the effects of burns, leaving women to carry the attacks with them permanently.

Chapter 4 discusses stigma, which is of primary interest in this endeavor. First, stigma theory is reviewed, then stigma theory is applied to facial disfigurement. Results of focus group discussions with over 20 severely disfigured Indian women are presented. Here, I'll posit theoretical ideas on the sociological origins of the Indian forms of disfigurement stigma. In short, it appears that this stigma is framed as threats to family roles and religious sensibilities. Stigma, it would seem, is the expression of fear and plays out in everyday life.

Finally, Chapter 5 provides a theoretical conclusion, bringing the themes presented in the first four chapters together (hopefully) into some sense of coherence. This study aims to explore how stigma is attached to disfigured women and how it relates to the sociocultural environment that produces it. While the stories about their lives as disfigured women are far from happy, many of the women interviewed for this study have learned to cope successfully with the way they are treated. Somehow they overcome the unbearable sadness, confusion, and dismay that come with the stigma and live fulfilled lives.

Doing disfigurement research is not easy. When I give lectures on disfigurement, my students are frequently stunned that such conditions exist in the world. They try to feel the pain that victims feel, and I am heartened by their displays of empathy and concern. I try to convey the same thoughts and feelings that I had when I began doing disfigurement studies many years ago. The first book I read about disfigurement was Lucy Grealy's *Autobiography of a Face*. Ms Grealy suffered from cancer in her face, and the disease and the treatments she was given left her permanently and severely disfigured. The quote below has stayed with me these many years and reminds me of the importance of studying disfigurement, particularly its social and psychological consequences, which by the way, are in no way the fault of disfigured people.

> I spent five years of my life being treated for cancer, but since then I've spent fifteen years being treated for nothing other than looking different from everyone else. It was the pain from that, from feeling ugly, that I always viewed as the great tragedy of my life. The fact that I had cancer seemed minor in comparison.

Socially speaking, the face is the most important part of our body. When faces are lost, lives rarely recover. I hope this book helps us to see the sources of this pain.

# 1

# Of Fire and Face

## The Stigma of Facial Burns

When you lose your face, you lose the whole world.

—Kanal Qayyam

The fate of our lives often rests in the hands of other people. For good, 'Think of all the beauty still left around you and be happy' (Anne Frank), or bad, 'Hell is other people' (Jean-Paul Sartre), our world is defined in relationship to other people. Both quotes reflect the sociological axiom that reality is socially constructed by the interconnectedness of people and the social forces they create. Be it for good or evil, we construct our world, giving it meaning, substance, and consequence, and it is people who create both the beauty that surrounds us and the evils that stalk and torment us.

These relationships occur neither in a vacuum nor randomly. Rules and ideas of value undergird social interaction and create boundaries of tolerance and acceptability. Some qualities or traits are highly prized by the social context of social interaction and are considered premium, while others that are negatively valued and are defined as taboo. The web of premium and taboo things is the basis of social and psychological life.

The difference between the premium and the taboo is the manner in which they are defined. All societies evaluate objects and ideas, and all social organizations have means for deciding upon the value of people. The criteria for such evaluations are numerous and are largely, if not exclusively, culturally sensitive. Different sociocultural settings evaluate human qualities in their own ideographic ways, judging people along criteria that history has created for them. We see other people and immediately begin to evaluate them according to social rules on defining characteristics such as age, sex, appearance, perceived status, race or ethnicity, and so forth, and these rules create either a pleasant or an unpleasant social experience.

The body, a person's corporeal presence, plays an important role in this equation. In our everyday surveillance of other people, we gaze at their bodies and consciously or unconsciously categorize them by types, each type having its own social meanings and relevance. The body is not the distinct physicality of humanness separated from the inner, existential, and inherently social human – mind and body duality is a myth. Instead the human body is tightly integrated with the social and psychological being. Bodies are, in fact, indistinguishable, and as Shilling states, the body is shaped, constrained, and, in a sense, invented by society. We observe bodies through the filters of our own psycho-socio-cultural contexts, and in doing so we have created the body as a social product with its own sense of social significance. Qualities of the body such as size and shape, skin color, hairstyle, and age all bear social meanings that decisively outweigh any biological relevance, and these social meanings vary from one group and individual to another.

As we scan and assess others' bodies, most of our attention is drawn to the face. It seems in our nature to evaluate the faces of others as attractive or unattractive, safe or threatening. We look into the eyes as the 'windows of the soul'. There is artistry in the face, and there is history. Many people even claim that the shape and movements of that single part of the body can predict the future. Facial movements fascinate us, and we are attracted to and repelled by them.

More than any other part of the body, the face provides important clues to understanding a social situation, and so we watch it carefully, our minds constantly decoding the messages we think we see. By watching others, we can develop clues as to whether a situation we come upon is dangerous, funny, or friendly. Faces, with their scores of muscles, are constantly in motion, representing and reacting to actions, emotions, and ideas. We watch and analyse how the oral complex, with its lips and surrounding muscles, and how the eyes, mysteriously recessed behind orbital bones and hidden behind eyelids and surrounded by brows and the nasal bridge, move up and down and side to side seemingly in rhythm to the moment. Our nose, the center of the visual target, ears, and forehead move more than we may realize, and these movements are noticed and are often perceived to send signals and cues as to the character of a person and what situation is happening.

Compared to other parts of the body, the face attracts the most attention because we often believe that facial appearance tells us everything we want or need to know about another person. We have expectations about the face. And style, as a concept, begins with the face. Faces should be kept clean, and, as cultural standards permit or require, they are adorned with jewelry, different patterns of facial hair, piercings, and colorations, all of which have social and situational meaning. Rightly or wrongly, facial actions are rife with social meaning; people define us by how our faces appear.

We are likely to judge pretty and handsome faces differently from ones we see as less attractive. The more eye-catching is another's face, the more we trust and feel safe. Faces that have trappings of wealth and authority – expensive hairstyles, well cared for skin, the 'right' skin color – exude confidence in others. Less attractive persons are likely evaluated more negatively. We may question the intelligence or motives of less attractive people, and if appearance does not fit social expectations in a particular situation, then others may question whether a particular person even belongs there. The face matters beyond simple sexual desirability, and facial appearance and facial motions are central features of everyday social interactions.

But what happens when the face is so severely scarred or distorted that we cannot recognize normal facial features or expressions? Do we see the person behind the normal face differently from the person with a disfigured face? How do people define an 'abnormal' face? Disfigurement changes the rules of usual, normative social engagement. Without doubt we understand or perceive or view severely disfigured individuals contrarily because of their appearance. The outward reaction to disfigurement may occur suddenly and even unconsciously, such as with a startle reflex, but we do react, and we certainly think about the disfigurement once the startle has ended, though we may not outwardly display anything further. We have to process it in our own minds and wonder how the disfigurement happened. Is this person a danger? Does this person have a contagion?

As we will see, the lives of severely disfigured people are distressed by how others treat them. For individuals whose appearance changes from normal to disfigured, the 'reality' of who they are, their own sense of personhood, literally changes along with their appearance. Other people alter their assessment of not only a disfigured person's appearance, but the person's character as well. Disfigured people are judged and evaluated differently from 'normals'. They essentially become different people. But why does that happen?

Changing perception of people who migrate from 'normal' to disfigured is not necessarily unexpected. Because sense of self and identity are neither static nor solely psychological processes, 'who people are' changes in general as social contexts evolve: definitions of groups and individuals are mutable. Sometimes these changes are slow paced, and on these occasions, perceptions of social groups change as part of the unfolding of global history. Civil rights movements lasting decades can alter out-groups' perceptions of ethnic groups and women, and awareness promotion campaigns affect sympathies for persons with disabilities, for instance. In another example, the shift to a postmodern culture in many parts of the world guides everyday thinking away from modernistic, typological conceptions of people and objects and toward fluid and contextual perceptions. Identity and feelings about others and ourselves relate to where we are in the history of the place we are nested. History indeed plays out in everyday life.

In other cases, definitions of reality change more abruptly, perhaps because of a singular act. We think differently of people who have been found guilty of a crime, for example, than we did before we knew about the conviction. People's actions create social consequences, and the definition of people changes not because of an act, but because of what follows an act. As W.I. Thomas famously said, 'If (people) define situations as real, they are real in their consequences'. How we frame what we see and feel constitutes reality, and this implies that what comes after an act can shape what the act actually is; that is, how it is defined and labeled. If Thomas is correct, there must be a set of social rules that guide how we define situations because it makes no sense to assume that social definitions are either reducible to psychologisms or are random.

This study is ultimately about how 'reality' can change for Indian women who become disfigured after having been set afire by their husbands. Although they may have survived, parts of these women's lives have been taken away because of how their world defines them after the assault. Reality and identity change for women whose husbands cause them to have scars rather than smooth skin, and lumps where noses, lips, and ears used to be. And the changes happen in the blink of an eye.

Many people find it hard to believe that such brutal attacks occur, especially within a family. Unfortunately it happens far more frequently than we may feel comfortable admitting. The women attacked this way often die a horrible and painful death. Survivors, as we will see, face tragedy and heartache in the conduct of their everyday lives because of their appearance. Stigmatized by society, many disfigured women have had their children and parents abandon them. More than just victims, these women are distrusted and feared because of their looks, and are frequently shunned. Many remain in pain, though their wounds may have healed. For some, simply being in the sunlight hurts their sensitive skin. Others have difficulty moving because of scar tissue. The lives of disfigured women tell us that the body is far more than the soul's façade.

The purpose of this study is to provide insight into the quality of life of Indian women who are disfigured by burn assaults and to gain a deeper understanding of the stigma that these women confront in everyday life. The stigma is more than just repulsion or a patriarchal-based rejection of women whose perceived sexual appeal is gone. Rather, an argument is posited that hostile reactions to women's disfigurement are rooted in the belief that an important facet of the moral basis of everyday life is challenged by disfigurement. Something other than perceived physical unattractiveness is operating because, as will be shown, people's objection to disfigured women runs deeper than the skin that is scarred and scored. The treatment these women face is rarely overtly sexualized. Most of the people who mistreat them are other women or men such as fathers and brothers who would have no sexual interest in them if they were not disfigured. There seems to be something buried in the ethos of the Indian mind that objects to disfigured women, and by examining the narratives of disfigured women we hope to find what those objections are.

## The Importance of the Human Face

The face is the epicenter of the human experience. The importance of the human face for personal and social identity, mate selection, and sexuality is unquestioned, and because we fret over our facial appearance, every year we spend billions of dollars on products and surgeries to improve, or at least make us think we are improving, our facial presentation. Perhaps our worry over our appearance is core to human existence. Evolutionary scientists have found that facial attractiveness is more important than any other physical feature in determining overall physical attractiveness (Currie and Little 2009), which may suggest that the face is a key species marker of genetic fitness and mate suitability. Not only is the face a clue to our sexuality, it is the physical feature that allows us to recognize each other and ourselves.

For most species in the animal kingdom, evolution has localized all of the senses except touch close to the brain. Vision, hearing, smell, and taste are centralized in one neurological and physiological command center, and the 'outlets' of these senses, the eyes, ears, nose, and mouth, shape the appearance of that area of the body into what we call the face. Eyes above, nose in the middle, and the mouth below, an arrangement known as first-order configuration, are constant features of the faces of human and nonhuman primates and monkeys and allows us (and primates and monkeys) to distinguish faces from other visual objects, that is, non-faces. Primates, including humans, and monkeys appear to have an innate attraction to faces, and the first-order facial recognition is the first step in specific facial recognition. Second-order facial configurations, which include coloration and slight differences in shape, provide the information necessary to individuate faces. Second-order patterns are recognized as individual specific and are the features that we integrate into a single perceptual whole (Parr 2011).

Recognizing second-order features is not unique to humans. Among other primates, faces vary, and individuals are capable of recognizing and differentiating each other. Although it is unclear how nonhuman primates make these distinctions, humans use holistic processing to recognize faces and distinguish one person from another. Our brains have developed neural and cognitive specializations that allow us to take the information presented by the specific areas of the face and integrate them into a singular perceptual whole. This process may account for why it is difficult to identify a familiar face if it is presented in a fragmented or unnaturalistic manner. As Parr (2011) states, recognizing faces is a difficult cognitive skill because of first-order configurations. All faces are arranged the same way. Nonetheless we are experts at noticing second-order arrangements and recognizing individual faces. From birth we are embedded in a facial world, and as we mature we become more adept at facial recognition.

Because we process faces holistically and each of us is embedded within a familiar socio-ethnic context, our expertise is strongest with faces within our own social groups. We sometimes struggle in processing faces of individuals in groups outside our own, often making it difficult to recognize and remember faces of individuals in other ethnic and racial groups. Our expertise, as it seems, is indeed constrained by familiarity.

In humans, because second-order differences are particularly discernable, each human face is physically unique. No two are truly identical. Even for monozygotic twins, each sibling's face is distinguishable, although the differences may be subtle and require keen observation to recognize. Given this uniqueness, our facial appearance is very personal and intimate.

Furthermore, second-order facial characteristics bear clues to gender, ethnic, and age identities, serving as symbolic markers of social status. In this regard faces are public objects. Our faces are the point of intersection between internal emotions and sentiments and the external, social world of relationships with other people. In other words, the face is the point of contact between our personal and public selves.

It is generally believed that some facial expressions, such as those connected to fear and that follow surprises, are involuntary and are taken as culturally universal. However, there is reason to believe that cultures interpret expressions differently and that cultures may impact what stimuli lead to a particular facial expression. We reflect on our faces and assess and judge them in reference to others' appearance and how we think others will evaluate our own appearance. In sum, the human face is a complicated and highly subjective part of the human body.

As the classical sociologist Georg Simmel contended, the face is a, if not *the*, measure of human significance. For him, the face is the outward expression of inward significance and is thus the conduit of a dialectic dance between concealing and revealing. Indeed the face is the playing field of most communication. Certainly oral communication occurs on the face, but so does a great amount of nonverbal and emotional expression. Although we know that facial expressions do not necessarily match internal motivations, and thus are not the same thing, there is a close connection between the two. The face can communicate emotions such as fear and anger, shame and embarrassment, and happiness and joy, and while we use our faces to send symbolic and emotional messages, we also deduce from others' expressions their moods and motivations. 'Reading' facial expressions provides critical information for understanding and defining a social situation as well as knowing how to channel our own emotions and cognitions, and imputing individual and social characteristics.

Conversely, we can also use the face to deceive others by concealing how we really feel with contrary facial expressions. The ability to give a disingenuous expression is a skill that can serve various ends. For example, some people are expert at hiding their true feelings or intentions in order to take advantage of a situation or person by using their 'poker face', a deliberately unemotional facial expression. Another example is that of flight attendants who use a soothing smile to console passengers anxious about flying, though they, the attendants, may not be in a particularly good mood or do not feel well during the flight (Hochschild 1983).

Since human facial expressions can be voluntary or manipulated reactions, Georg Hegel, the great German philosopher, believed that facial expressions are actions unto themselves, existing separately from internal emotions and character. The face therefore provides its own text and becomes a part of a social interaction, just as any other social action. And just like any behavior, facial expressions fall within social contextual parameters. They are situational and have cultural relevance and meaning.

Hegel's position contradicts the historically Western tradition of physiognomy, the belief that a person's character and personality could be deduced and understood by assessing facial features. Dating back to the Greeks and Romans, beauty was equated with perfection, love, and virtue: Beauty was found in mathematics, nature, as well as the human physique. The opposite was also considered true: Certain physical qualities that were defined as ugliness were linked to the lack of virtue and criminality. As late as the 19th and 20th centuries, theories that body types, including facial features, predicted and caused criminal behavior and certain personality traits were proffered at the highest levels of scientific discourse. The well-known Cesare Lombroso, for example, contended that criminal behavior was essentially a consequence of backward evolution. Criminals were genetically regressed subhumans incapable of following the expectations of civilized, that is, advanced European society, which held characteristics of earlier, more primitive forms of human ancestry. His so-called criminaloid type, the 'born criminal', could be identified by facial features such as low foreheads, asymmetrical faces and craniums, broad noses, forehead wrinkles, receding hairlines, and other body features. William Sheldon, writing in the 1940s, contended that body types were associated with temperaments. His three somatotypes were the ectomorph (a slim, lean body), mesomorph (large bones, solid torso, muscular), and endomorph (wide hips and frame, better able to retain fat), were believed to correspond to particular characterological traits and dispositions. We now know that 'society' stereotypes people with various physical traits, rather than the traits causing the characterizations of them, and theories such as Lombroso's primitive notions of genetics and Sheldon's somatotype psychology have been dismissed as lacking the reliability and validity necessary to sustain the ideas.

Faces have subjective meaning beyond banal sexual attractiveness. We project onto other individuals' appearances the stories of their lives, which as a projection really tells us more about ourselves. As Trachtenberg (2000) states, others' faces trigger our memories, excite speculation, and reveal thoughts about the past and future. Faces possess their own subjective narratives. An easy exercise to see this is to dwell on a portrait, either painted, sculpted, or photographed. When we do this, we 'see' a life, perhaps a latent life that becomes animated by the ideals and traits we extract from it (it could be argued that we are projecting those qualities onto the portrait). We assess the portrait, not necessarily according to the mechanics of the artist's creativity and intent, but as an expression of qualities and histories that are uniquely human. We look at portraits, such as the Mona Lisa, and see a person within a social situation.

These judgments have real life implications. For decades, research has shown that physical appearance plays an important role in how people fare in social situations. We know, for example, that an appearance judged as more beautiful and ideal influences income, career mobility, and perceived competence (Biddle and Hamermesh 1998; Gehrsitz 2014; Hamermesh and Biddle 1994; Harper 2000; Judge et al. 2009; Mobius and Rosenblat 2006).

These findings support Goffman's (1963) notions that certain 'presentations of self', or self-images, are expected to match social situations, and consequently, we must manage our social image vis-à-vis the expectations of the situation in which we find ourselves. We must create an image that is in harmony with the expectations of the situation, which are constructions of the rules of the group and norms governing the particular social context. Usually we take an expressive posture that is legitimate, according to Goffman, and we must maintain that image for the situation to continue. The image we present is not freely selected; rather, it is a choice selected from a socially prescribed set of available options – options that are morally proper, given the rules. We use a sad face in situations of sorrow, for example. To show a smile, at a funeral for instance, is considered most inappropriate.

When we present improper impressions, or what Goffman calls a 'wrong face', our social worth cannot easily be integrated into the social situation, and we cannot take an expected or morally appropriate position in that situation. We cannot, using Goffman's words, weave 'ourselves into the expressive fabric of the occasion' (1963: 7). We are excluded and rejected, and often left to feel ashamed and inadequate, and we are most certainly judged. The criteria on which we are evaluated are a complex of norms and values that often evoke the deepest moral sentiments of the society. These rules are often so deeply ingrained in our psyches that we think of them as natural and even genetic. Thus, if an individual presents the wrong 'face', then he or she is out of sync with the situation and judged on the severity of the inconsistency.

To put it all together, the human face is so intertwined with identity that the face and sense of self are often considered inseparable (Macgregor 1951). As Synnott (1989: 607) states, the face is the 'prime symbol of the self'. For Simmel (1964), therefore, the face is 'the spirit of society', the characterization of both individual and societal essence, intention, and organization.

## Severe Disfigurement

Further evidence of the importance of the face in human life are the social and psychological outcomes of a severely disfigured face; a face that via trauma, congenital anomaly, or disease is rendered so different from a culture's norm of standard appearance as to make disfigured persons themselves social anomalies. For many severely disfigured faces because of injuries to skin, muscles, bones, and other tissues, the first-order configuration of the face is compromised and second-order patterns are unrecognizable. Standards of both humanness and beauty are violated in severely disfigured faces, and the usual methods of carrying out our innate ability to focus on faces are disrupted. We have trouble processing disfigured faces because they are so different from 'normal' faces of high familiarity. We find it hard to engage them holistically perhaps because the disfigurement interferes with our ability to extract information. In other words, disfigured faces do not give us the social cues that we rely upon to make sense of social and emotional situations.

Severely disfigured faces are often incapable of 'normal' expressiveness and thus are unable to transmit those cues that help define social situations and interactions. The inability to express emotions or fully engage in a conversation with appropriate facial expressions marks the disfigured person as different, perhaps a little too different for inclusion in routine social life. A disfigured person is *always* presenting the 'wrong face' and the rules of situational interaction are curiously and automatically broken. The presentation of the self, which is constantly managed in part by facial expression and appearance, now must include the scars of disfigurement to perhaps the part of the body that has the most impact on social image. Disfigured people cannot easily take the expected social posture required of a social situation not because of functionality, but because the disfigurement itself seems to be a violation of the social rules governing impression management.

The face becomes disfigured persons' defining feature and marks what symbolic interaction theory calls the master (i.e. dominant) social status (Furr et al. 2007). One's master status dominates all other characteristics a person may hold and essentially represents who that person is. Disfigurement overrides other traits or qualities a person holds and elicits treatment different from that which non-disfigured people encounter. Scores of studies in the United States and United Kingdom have identified the many injurious psychosocial *sequelae* of severe disfigurement and concluded that severely disfigured people are deeply stigmatized.

When people see a disfigured face, what, in fact, do they 'see'? What thoughts, cues, or ideas are projected? What situation is perceived? In Hegel's reckoning, what is the social act embodied in the disfigured face? As disfigured people will quickly attest, others respond to them initially with a startled response. Upon seeing them, others either quickly look away or stare and then more often than not will engage in an approach-and-avoidance dance in which the 'normal' person will approach the disfigured person with trepidation and anxiety or will take steps to avoid the disfigured person altogether. Sometimes people ask intrusive, personal questions about the disfigured person's unusual appearance, and others may make insulting or ridiculing comments. Disfigured persons say that these responses are so common that they are predictable and expected. Eventually disfigured persons learn to avoid interacting with other people for fear of the punishing nature of the contact. Clearly something is communicated or insinuated by the disfigured face. This face has meaning. It is a social act: two people are required to create disfigurement, the person whose face has been altered and a second person to interpret that face as disfigured and not normal. At this point, all we know is that the disfigured face is stigmatized, which means that it has been labeled as discrediting, causing disfigured persons to lose something socially.

Although the stigma attached to disfigurement is known to be harsh, it is not fully understood, particularly in a cross-cultural context. Little research has been conducted on the lives of disfigured persons in India, and what is especially unclear is how severe facial disfigurement is interpreted in India where the rules guiding the management of facial expressions and gender-informed definitions of face and body differ from Western norms.

## Of Fire and Face In India

*Fire:* Attack by acid and fire is a crime of severe magnitude that results in death at worst and permanent disfiguration at least. For survivors, there is neither full recovery nor a return to normalcy. Yet despite its brutality and the media attention the crime has received of late, relatively little is known about those who attack women in this manner. No study of perpetrators has yet been conducted to understand their motivations, emotional state, or ideas about women and male entitlements. We know the circumstances of burn assaults, which will be explored in a latter chapter. However, we cannot identify the psychosocial characteristics of a person who attacks with acid and fire or the specific situations in which the attack is more likely to occur. In other words, we lack the data and theory that would allow us to profile the burn attacker.

Nevertheless, we can make several assumptions about the nature of burn attacks, assumptions that help contextualize the stigma attached to the victims. First, acid and thermal face burning is an attack of extremely deep-seated anger that transcends the interpersonal conflict the perpetrator and victim may have had. It is a very personal and intimate crime in which the intent is clearly not simply to harm or punish, but to damage the totality of victims' lives. By rendering victims, quite literally, faceless in the crowd, the goal is not only to destroy the face, but to ruin victims' identity and social location. Fire and acid are weapons of intense passions, regardless of how irrational the motivations to burn someone may appear, and the emotions are vitriolic and intensely personal.

A second axiom guiding this study is that fire holds powerful symbolic meaning in Indian cultures. South Asian clerics have taught for millennia that fire is a powerful medium for reaching the gods and purification. These themes are certainly not unique to Hinduism, but few contemporary religions place as much emphasis on fire as do Hindus.

Fire has potent magical qualities and power in the Hindu epistemology and is an instrument of practical everyday change and problem solving. When accompanied by the correct prayer or mantra, fire or just a single flame can facilitate wish and goal fulfillment and transform that which is impure and material to clean and spiritual. Fire sacrifice of flowers and foodstuffs, for example, is an age-old practice of appealing to Vishnu to grant requests. The flame's power sends the offerings directly to the mouth of Vishnu and appeases the god, which makes granting the worshippers' prayers more likely.

To Westerners, cremation is perhaps the most well-known Hindu fire ritual. Core to Hindu beliefs, cremation is necessary to release the 'pure' soul from the 'impure' body upon the latter's death. From the Sri Isha Upanishad:

> Let this temporary body be burned to ashes, and let the air of life be merged with the totality of air. Now, O' my Lord, please remember all my sacrifices, and because You are the ultimate beneficiary, please remember all that I have done for You.
>
> O' my Lord, powerful as the fire, omnipotent one, now I do offer You all obeisances and fall at Your feet on the ground. O my Lord, please lead me on the right path to reach You, and since You know all that I have done in the past, please free me from the reactions to my past sins, so that there will be no hindrance to my progress.

The pure eternal soul is freed from the temporal and polluted body and returns to heaven through the vehicle of fire and the rituals performed by priests and the deceased's eldest son. Thus, 'progress' toward nirvana is assured.

Perhaps it is a macabre symbolic need or urge to cleanse the world of perceived impurity that prompts men to attempt to end the lives of their wives by setting them on fire. As shall be seen, women who are burned by their husbands are highly likely to have experienced physical and emotional abuse in their marriages. Prior to the burns and because of this abuse, their lives were dreary and painful. In light of this abuse, it is feasible that these husbands found their wives disappointing, hence the need to punish, torture, and kill them. Setting their wives on fire perhaps is an unconscious ritualistic way of sloughing off unclean and unwanted objects that are not satisfactorily living up to some set of expectations. Annihilating that object with fire must carry special meaning, given that there are many far less severe ways to end a marriage or solve a problem.

On an everyday and mundane level, fire and acid are valued because of their cleaning properties. Fire sterilizes sullied surfaces and is widely used to 'clean' agricultural fields of unwanted plants or the remains of the previous crop. Acid, as mentioned earlier, is an ordinary though potent cleansing agent that sears away grime and filth. In sum, burning maintains sacred and secular, practical and magical virtues that can purify anything from an infected needle to a soiled toilet to a sinner's body.

*Face:* In traditional India, women are subject to the demands of a strict patriarchy in which their rights are limited and prospects for a life outcome other than that prescribed by the patriarchy are a near impossibility. Women's value, in most of Indian society, is purely instrumental and largely confined to sexuality, maintaining a household, and producing sons. Marriages are usually arranged, negotiated by parents and influenced by other family elders and astrological consults through the ancient practice of *gotra*, and when a woman is married, she leaves her family of origin and joins her husband's and the hierarchy of his household, which typically requires submission to her mother-in-law.

Caste accounts for most differences in life chances in India, but all castes have one thing in common. As a young woman's parents bargain her away, parents in all castes share one asset – their daughters' appearance. Shrewd parents of particularly attractive daughters will use that asset to improve not only their daughter's social status, but also their own, as parents rely on their children's economic good fortunes for support in their elderly years. The demands of caste dictate endogamy; however, women can move up in status, albeit only in small measures, if she proves to have personal (i.e. physical) qualities that a man and his family cannot attain within their own caste. The more beautiful a woman is, the more desirable she becomes and the greater the perception that she will fulfill the essential qualities demanded of women.

Therefore, a woman's face is her most important quality; it is her native wealth. Of course, the significance of female physical attraction is not unique to India and South Asian cultures and history, and the status of women as more than pure objects is slowly improving, though it is still poor compared to other global democracies. In India, however, the dominance of physical attributes over all others has remained deeply embedded in the culture into the 21st century. Physical reductionism, which for our purposes includes both appearance and bearing sons, seems to have persisted in ranking women's worth in everyday Indian society, trumping intellectual powers, emotional companionship, and the mutually reinforcing personal growth among partners.

Perhaps this meaning of the face is perpetuated in India because it is reinforced by the particularly special meanings placed on the head in general in Hindu cosmology. While the head and face are recognized as important for basic human functioning, thc *Mahanarayana Upanishad* assigns them special significance by stating that one honors the deity with the head. The forehead, for example, bears the *bindi* (*tilaka* in Sanskrit), the sign of the divine eye or the third eye of spiritual awakening and consciousness. Whereas physical eyes, the eyeballs, look outward toward the material world, the third eye is metaphysical and looks inward into the spiritual domain. And though *bindis* are now regularly worn cosmetically and are often quite stylish, the traditional *bindi* is a sign of piety and love, and through color variations, they can designate marital status or caste position, ranks that carry social and religious weight.

The crown of the head is the point on the body of greatest religious significance in traditional Hindu spiritualism. The ancients believed that a channel (*susumna*) ran through the body to the top of the head, and upon death it is via this pathway that the soul leaves the body to attain immortality (*Katharudra Upandishad*; Brown 1921/2016). Through *susumna*, and other channels, flows *prana*, the life force or vital energy of life. At certain points, *chakras*, which are nodes of *prana* energy, are found vertically and hierarchically throughout the body. Each *chakra* is associated with a quality, emotion, or value. The lower *chakras*, those found in the ankles and feet, have the most negative connotations. *Rasatala chakra* (ankles) is connected to base animal instincts, while the foot *chakra* is associated with a state without consciousness (*mahatala*). The bottom of the feet is the lowest, least pure part of the body. The *patala chakra*, centered in the soles of the feet, marks the borderline of hell (*naraka*). *Patala chakra* constitutes the realm of hatred, murder, and sadism, and its ruling forces are malice and destruction. Traditional Hindu mores discourage showing the bottoms of the feet, especially to individuals of a higher caste position.

On the other hand, at the crown of the head, is the *sahasrara* chakra. The crown *chakra* is the state of pure consciousness, the highest form of being. When *prana* is raised to the *sahasrara chakra* through moral living and deep meditation, nirvana or heaven is reached. The head, therefore, is the most sacred region of the body, the point of contact not with hell, but with purity and true, enlightened consciousness. Whereas in the *patala* region lays the consequences of the misdeeds from previous lives, *sahasrara* is the essence of goodness and godliness. It is the site of approaching god, not *naraka*.

Perhaps because of the combination of the face being so close to the *susumna* and the *chakra* path of holiness while holding unique human functional significance, the meaning of the face is deeply embedded in the Indian consciousness in ways that may differ from other cultures. Many gods within the pantheon of Hindu deities have multiple heads. The god of creation, Purusa, for example, has a thousand heads, which the *Mudgala Upanishad* interprets as an infinity of heads. Brahma, the creator god, has four faces. Other gods are occasionally presented with multiple faces that represent different aspects of character.

It is difficult to determine the degree to which these material and corporeal depictions of deities have direct influence on a person's behavior. These divine images do, however, represent a cultural influence, a baseline, if you will, of values and social definitions of goodness, badness, and expectations. Therefore, the faces of Hindu gods contribute to the way in which human faces are defined and understood. The gods represent ideals, and humans are measured against them, and that holds for both behavior and appearance. Consequently, the face has deep significance in Indian sensibilities as a revealer of intent, power, and goodness. To lose the face is indeed to lose the world.

A final axiom guiding our understanding of burn attacks concerns the status of women in Indian society, which, being quite low compared to that of men, makes them vulnerable to violence and seemingly disposable. More specifically, women in India are typically reduced to a state of being 'essentialized'; that is, women are assumed to share a fundamental nature that gives rise to their observable characteristics. One consequence of gender essentialization, as Prentice and Miller (2006: 130) state, is that 'any one woman can stand in for the category', which means that all women are essentially the same person and are therefore interchangeable. As will be discussed in Chapter 2, essentialization lends Indian women to becoming subject to a number of social disadvantages such as domestic and political violence, political disenfranchisement, and unequal access to education, economic opportunities, and health.

While women's status is largely that of a second-class citizen, the roles women play are in many ways the glue that bonds all social life in India. The family, which is the basic unit of culture and identity, is the social space in which most of women's supposed essential traits play out and are prized. The caste system imposes strict rules on who marries whom, making caste endogamy highly important, and determines a household's division of labor. A goal of traditional Indian women is to become the senior wife, the wife of the family's patriarch. The elder mother-in-law commands the household, ordering about daughters-in-law and, in more well-to-do homes, servants. A woman can achieve this position by having sons.

The ability to produce sons is another attribute of the successful essentialized woman. Son preference is very strong in India because of the need for sons' labor to support the family, the opportunity to bring in daughters-in-law for domestic work and grandsons, and to conduct important funeral rituals for parents. In much of Indian culture, not producing at least one son is a curse for women. Being sonless often leads to shame, embarrassment, and ridicule in women's families and immediate community. Men without sons are often dishonored.

Lastly, the essentialized woman is defined by labor in service to husbands (cooking, cleaning, child-raising, etc.). Women are expected to be flawless cooks and caregivers and loyal and ever-ready sexual partners. In addition to their domestic labor, women, especially those in or near poverty, are expected to add cash income to the family's coffers.

A woman disfigured before marriage or abandoned by her husband cannot achieve the basic essentialized female self as culturally defined and therefore threatens the cultural and social order that hinges upon women's attractiveness and labor. Opportunities for hypergamy are beyond reach, and no amount of dowry will make disfigured women appealing. They remain burdens on their parents, which means that they likely will not provide old-age social security or much-desired grandchildren. Women who fail to live up to traditional essentialist expectations or are perceived to fail are reduced to near nothingness.

## Conclusion

Most studies on stigma focus on its effects on victims' individual adjustment and well-being. Few stigma researchers, and none in the disfigurement literature, have looked at the stigmatizers, a point of neglect hopefully informed by the current research strategy that included interviews with disfigured women in India. The study is designed to achieve two goals. The first and primary aim is to understand sociologically the stigma ascribed to disfigured women in India. A second goal is that perhaps by studying stigma, we might also gain additional insights into why women are burned in the first place.

Gendered violence against women is found in most, if not all, societies, but burning women is not. It happens in only a few societies, mostly in South Asia, that have cultures grounded in principles of extreme male privilege. Burning is torturous and permanent and essentially destroys women's traditional 'value', which of course is largely based on her appearance and sexuality. How are South Asian patriarchies, particularly India, distinguished from other male-dominated social systems around the world where the treatment of women is less vitriolic?

The goal of this study is to fuse the themes of the significance of fire, the meaning of the human face, and violence toward women into an understanding of the meanings of facial disfigurement in India through the analysis of stigma. The study proposes that severe disfigurement in India is not just a transgression against the body, but also a blemish on the character of the disfigured person. The study will attempt to make sociological sense of the stories of Indian women who have been disfigured by their husbands who, through attacks by fire, sought to dislodge these women from their own lives.

To follow through on Satre's proposition, if 'hell is other people', for disfigured women in India, stigma is hell's *modus operandi*.

# 2

# The Meaning of Gender in India

> Raising a daughter is like watering your neighbor's garden.
>
> —Indian saying

In 1904, Herbert Compton wrote: 'Ladies first', we say in the West; in the East (meaning India) it is Ladies last'. Compton was a British military officer who was stationed in colonial India and who later became an attorney, eventually serving as a judge in Mumbai, Chennai, and Kolkata. Though looking at India through colonial and highly ethnocentric lenses, he took notice of the gender disparity that characterized traditional Indian society and continues to be a distinguishing feature of the society into the 21st century. Of course, women's rights and lived existence were not much better in Britain in the 19th and early 20th centuries than they were in India, and the colonists, as many have argued, aggravated or worsened gender inequalities in the subcontinent. However, Compton did sense a different kind of relationship between men and women in India from that which occurred in England. His observation proved prophetic. Women's entitlements and opportunities have expanded greatly in Western societies since 1900, but in India, economic and political disparity and high incidences of gendered violence, female infanticide, and sex-selective abortion remain central to the social order.

Here are a few statistical 'snapshots' that, taken together, fashion an overall image of the differences between the lives of Indian men and women. India ranks 130 of 155 countries on the United Nations Human Development Scale and among the lowest countries on the Gender Inequality Index. Government of India indicators show that women fare poorly on most all social well-being measures when compared to men. Women's labor force participation is about half that of men's, and they are more vulnerable to malnutrition than boys and men. Women are grossly underrepresented in corporate and government leadership positions. For example, fewer than 10 per cent of High Court and Supreme Court judges are women, which is interesting given that fewer than 15 per cent of domestic violence cases in which women are victims are prosecuted and only about 9 per cent are convicted, according to the Government of India national statistics in 2012. The social disparities between men and women are numerous and not spurious. The picture is not pretty.

Because of the stark differences in the overall quality of life between women and men, scholars and activists are tempted to assume that the patriarchy, which is indeed core to Indian social organization, acts upon all women the same, creating a singular 'female type'. Rather, because women's lives in India, as elsewhere, are tempered and molded by caste, religion, family dynamics, education and other factors (Berreman 1992), we must not think of or specify a singular 'Indian woman'. These status markers impact virtually all indicators of women's quality of life; age at marriage and first pregnancy, overall fertility, and risk of violence are all subject to intersections with other status markers. As example, despite being subjected to the same patriarchal system, wealthy high caste women live quite different lives from impoverished low caste women. With wealth and caste come social privileges impossible for poor woman to imagine. Access to education, health care, rewarding economic activities, and basic human services such as clean water and sanitation enhances the lives of the wealthy.

Nonetheless, the experience of women is not parallel to that of men, even when comparing them within comparable castes or other status positions in India. The purpose of this chapter, therefore, is to explore these differences to help us better understand how and why women are more likely to be burned by men and suffer the stigma they experience afterwards. This chapter will review the quality of life of women in India from the perspective that everyday life is regulated by the social construction of gender and that the meanings of gender and sex have real and substantial life consequences. This chapter seeks to illustrate the psychosocial landscape in which both formal and informal society seemingly condone violence against women, a crime that often goes unpunished, and govern how women are treated after violence has disfigured them. As Jejeebhoy and Cook (1997) have averred, violence against women is so common that it seems to be a cultural norm and should be considered a part of womanhood. If violence is normative, then the consequences of violence are as well.

## Social Construction and Essentialism

Any theoretical guide attempting to explain gender relationships in India, or anywhere for that matter, must be grounded in the social definition of the body, which redirects the meaning of socially neutral males and females into socially constructed boys and girls and men and women. Gendering the biologic casts the fate of individuals at birth, if not before; as Simone de Beauvoir (1973: 301) famously said, 'One is not born, but rather becomes, a woman'. In this view, anatomy is not destiny, but the social meanings of anatomy are.

### *The Essentialized Woman*

Debate continues over gender essentialism, of whether or not there are foundational, physiological differences between males and females that guide and direct the psychological and behavior orientation of individuals and the gendered structure of the social order. Essentialism, therefore, is arguing the presence of a metaphorical 'gender gene' that implies a biological determinism to temperament, ability, values, emotions, and social position. Essentialism can further suggest universal claims about all women – that all women possess common qualities, reactions, and experiences.

At the beginning of this chapter, we noted that the experiences of women in any one society can vary to a great degree. Social class and caste alone account for many differences among women within a society, making it difficult to recognize any similarities in the lives of the rich and poor within the same society; how they experience life is in many ways unalike and shares little in common. Alison Stone is correct that 'theories that claim that all women share a common social position will always be falsely overgeneralized' (2007: 147).[1]

I prefer to think of gender essentialism as a verb: to essentialize the 'other'. It means to create and impose the idea that men and women have unique and intrinsic physiological characteristics that imply and influence social and psychological traits, aptitudes, propensities, and capabilities. Despite the absence of meaningful biological evidence that would account for such essentialist conclusions, some segments of virtually all societies will define males and females *as if* they are substantially disparate and even contradictory to one another in their humanness.

Therefore, essentialism exists as a political and socially defining ideology that differentially and externally guides the life chances and behavioral expectations of males and females. While we don't yet know if there is an inherent 'femaleness' or 'maleness' in humans, given, in fact, evidence to the contrary, we can state that essentialism is a socially constructed artifact of a power structure that politically and economically enables men but restricts opportunities for women. Political essentialism contends that women are unfit or unable to perform the duties and roles of power and leadership, roles that are largely awarded to men. Too emotional, too ignorant, too unreliable, women subjected to essentialist beliefs are defined as inapt in the 'man's world'. In this ideology, women don't have the wherewithal to compete or meet the physical and intellectual demands asked of males. Essentialist qualities may or may not be inherent, but they are certainly imposed.

Essentialist reductionism is necessary to a patriarchal power system because it provides the justification for gender inequality. As Charlotte Witt contends, 'gender has a normative priority in relation to other social roles in an individual's social agency' (2011: 79). This hints at the idea that essentialism is a socially constructed, yet seemingly paradoxical proposition: that in the absence of valid evidence of inherent differences, 'society' says there are. As Witt continues, 'gender is the central thread that connects, organizes, and defines our social existence' (2011: 106). Essentialism is important in a patriarchy as it provides the means for stratifying the sexes and creates a division of experience that crosses all social lines and enters into all aspects of social life. Where biology fails to account for gender, essentialism fills the gap and 'explains' why women are unequal to men.

Perceptions of the body create the gendered body and the subsequent social space in which women and men live their everyday lives. These social forces have their own weight and continuity, evolving and reproducing over time and from one generation to the next. These forces are supported by acts of power and are organized as social institutions. In turn, they are legitimized by internalizing the precepts of patriarchy and are exerted in the everyday space of social life. The basic tenets of essentialist beliefs become 'natural' and undisputed facts of life.

That women of all castes continue to struggle for opportunities in ways that men do not is example of the long-held feminist notion that social inequalities are structured by perceptions of the natural body (Shilling 2005). More to the point, Foucault argued that the body, or physical self, is an unfixed, malleable object in which power is invested; power controls individuals through the conception of the human body. The very idea of 'the body' is produced by social forces that identify bodies as having certain social meanings, regardless of any biological constitution, limitation, or proclivity. The body, therefore, is a biological phenomenon that has a sociological definition, and as a social object, it is endowed with social meaning, complete with definitions of social opportunities and limits.

As 'society' recognizes the biological sex, it simultaneously recognizes the limits of acceptable behavior for that sex. The female body is therefore defined as inherently and differently social and political from the male body. Hence gender is socially constructed, and cultural values and social precepts bind men and women into demands of conformity, aided by law, religion, and customs, which allow a tolerated range of acceptability that is wider for men than women. These gender positions, subsequently, are stratified and ranked, implying a perception of unequal value and worth and are loci of dominance and subordinance.

Bourdieu's 'habitus' is a particularly useful concept for understanding the relationship between social position and personal characteristics. Wacquant correctly interprets habitus as 'the way society becomes deposited in persons in the form of lasting dispositions, or trained capacities and structured propensities to think, feel and act in determinant ways, which then guide them' (2005: 316). For Bourdieu (1977), behavior, tastes, personal styles, and even emotions are developed in relationship to everyday practices, which he conceived as modes of behavior conditioned by individuals' position or relationship to other modes or dispositions of behavior, values, styles, and so forth.[2] Dispositions form through encountering others and become what Bourdieu called 'a sense of the game' (Bourdieu and Wacquant 1992). How one acts and thinks is a practical response, sometimes rational and sometimes intuitive, to power relations, symbolic meanings, and the instrumental necessities of everyday life.

With this formula, it's no wonder that higher social class positions have a positive influence on intellectual flexibility, a preference for self-direction over conformity (Kohn and Schooler 1973) and a heightened sense of self-efficacy (Gecas 1989), which is the degree that individuals believe in their own ability to complete tasks, reach goals, and control their own lives. For higher class and caste individuals, these qualities influence life outcomes by enabling achievement. Success for lower caste people, which in this case means women in their relationship to men, is rooted in obeyance, following the norms of gendered relationships that define women's place in the social order, and also the rewards of being the 'good woman'. The 'good woman', of course, is the woman who follows the rules and minds her place.

Structured subservience demands the individual emotional and behavioral wherewithal to survive that subservience. At the other end of the spectrum, power teases out and requires personality qualities that allow the holder of power to dominate others. Those in dominant positions play the role of the power positions, exercising command and executive functions in families and intersexual relationships. There is a sense of command and authority that is self-rewarding to men, regardless of caste or class. Privilege, simply expressed, feels good.

Of course, many if not most holders of dominance and authority positions are not despotic beasts; yet few wielders of power, authority, and wealth voluntarily relinquish their position of advantage out of guilt or empathy for the subjects of their power. Men, as a class, have a structural interest in maintaining male privilege and that requires them to control subordination. Ideological requisites that lessen female value informs this inequality, and formal and informal norms of control, such as rules that minimize women's inheritance, dynamics that reproduce higher illiteracy rates for girls and women, and a disproportional exposure to interpersonal and domestic violence, all intersect to perpetuate gender differences and maintain the boundaries separating the sexes. An understanding of those men who commit violence against women must begin not with the psychology of any individual perpetrator, but with the material, structured social relationships that govern gender relations. Violence against women, to use C. Wright Mills' famous equation, is a public issue rather than a personal trouble. A victim of violence certainly feels pain and heartbreak on a personal basis, but to comprehend violence that occurs in broad-sweeping social patterns such as intimate partner violence, we must look at the organized configuration of how men and women relate to each other.

## Status of Women

Despite substantial improvements in women's lives in India over the last couple of decades, the well-being of women in comparison to men falls far short of equality with men. In terms of health and education, political empowerment, and equal protection of the law, women's place in society fails to reach those ranks that are enjoyed by men.

Women in subcontinental cultures have not always suffered the level of inequality they face in more contemporary times, however. Many historians believe that in the formative years of the cultures of South Asia, women enjoyed relatively equal status to that of men. In the early Vedic Age, roughly 2000 BCE to 500 BCE, it is supposed that women's position in society was not hampered by the many restrictions that would eventually evolve into the modern patriarchy. Although the early Vedic period was definitely male dominated, women had certain rights and privileges that they would lose over the course of time. In the days before female feticide and sati, prayers asking for healthy and intelligent daughters were proffered routinely, and girls received an education similar to that of boys. Contrary to later times, women scholars in Vedic India contributed to knowledge. What's more, women could choose their marital partners, and their mere presence did not pose obstacles to religious rituals.

Despite these relative advantages in status, most historians agree that women and men in the early Vedic Age encountered each other within the context of gendered rules that sought to control women's sexuality, and though women worked side by side with men in their agricultural economies, women's sexuality was protected, prized, and controlled by men in a complex web of structured gendered relationships. Men, however, were not comparably defined and controlled.

To make a complicated history extraordinarily brief,[3] with the beginnings of greater technological and social complexity[4] and wealth, the social organization of the cultures of India evolved around the formation of caste groups that had sharp boundaries and clearly defined rights and privileges. Writings from the Vedic period give us some measure of what life was like, or at least intended to be. From circa 1500 BCE to several centuries into the Common Era, religious epics and sacred hymns, stories, and texts, such as the *Rigveda*, *Mahabharata*, and *Ramayana*, were composed and compiled. These classical writings not only spelled out Hindu cosmology, but also narrated codes of conduct, some of which pertained to the interaction between women and men. Knowledge of these great works spread throughout the region, and the ideas they contained became the foundational norms and values of social behavior. As the great B.R. Ambedkar and others have stated, the early Hindu literature is responsible for many of the ideas that contributed to the persistent and modern subjugation of women (George 2005).

For example, the *Ramayana*, the famous Sanskrit epic poem dating back to about 400 BCE, is believed by most Indians to have had a profound impact on the psyche of Indian men and women. The story is well-known throughout India and is sometimes colloquially referred to as the History of India. Part of the plot is that Rama's wife, Sita, who is beautiful and of incomparable virtue, is kidnapped by the evil Ravana. Eventually Rama rescues his queen, but he begins to worry that she has not been faithful to him during her many years of capture. To relieve his anxiety, he subjects Sita to a public test, a trial by fire in which she is made to enter a conflagration: if she emerges unburned, his wife's fidelity is confirmed. And this is exactly what happens. Sita was indeed true and faithful to Rama, verifying her loyalty to her husband despite great adversity and hardship.

One of the important themes of the *Ramayana* is its portrayal of the expectations of the ideal man and the ideal woman. As everyone in India knows, Sita is the image of the exalted female spirit. She is the epitome of the perfect woman, the exemplar, the 'ideal type' about which all girls and women are taught to aspire and are evaluated. Sita is the essential female character: she is glorified for her loyalty to her husband

and is revered as a Divine Mother. Sita suffered for her husband, but did not complain, as she is unselfish, self-effacing, and pure of heart.

Denial of the self in order to serve husbands and sons lies at the very core of patriarchy, and it is this leitmotif that has guided the socialization of Indian girls and women for tens of centuries. Girls aspire to be Sita; men expect to have Sita as their wives. The *Ramayana* has had a long and deep impact on the definition of Indian women's sense of self. As Anju P. Bhargava (2000) has said: 'Sita is an integral part of our (Indian women's) psyche. At every stage of an Indian woman's life her name is invoked'.

Another of the more important of these time-honored texts is the Law of Manu, known as the *Manusmriti*, which was written circa 200 BCE to 200 CE. Though it is likely that the *Manusmriti* drew from existing texts and reflects 'a crystallization of an accumulated knowledge' of ancient India (Olivelle 2005: 24–25), the dissemination of the *Manusmriti* is important in the history of India in that it organized the moral underpinnings of Hindu cultures. Extolling the virtues of civility, the *Manusmriti* set the cosmology of Hindu life by providing an explanation of the origins of the world and shaped the standards of ordinary morality. The code, for example, describes the virtues of vegetarianism and prohibits lying and stealing, and it outlines the rules of conduct for the four *varnas*, the basic or foundational divisions of Hindu social organization. The *Manusmriti* was never used as a codified system of laws, and its influence actually may have been stronger on the British Orientalists who helped shape Indian law during colonial times (Lal 2013; Kishwar 1994); nevertheless, it provides an excellent reflection of everyday life, or at least what everyday life should be, in the eyes of an ancient, but conservative India, and became a fundamental text upon which laws were based.

Of pertinent significance is the Law of Manu's legalistic rendering of the rules that govern the relationships between women and men, instructions that clearly relegate women to a subservient, dependent position, without any access to civil liberties and self-determination. For example, the code states

> Girls are supposed to be in the custody of their father when they are children, women must be under the custody of their husband when married and under the custody of her son as widows. In no circumstances is she allowed to assert herself independently. (5/151)

and

> It is the duty of all husbands to exert total control over their wives. Even physically weak husbands must strive to control their wives. (9/6)

and

> Men may be lacking virtue, be sexual perverts, immoral and devoid any good qualities, and yet women must constantly worship and serve their husbands. (5/157)

If Olivelle is correct that the *Manusmriti* represents what life was and what it should be according to cultural leaders of the day, then we can assume that gender was constructed in such a way that the lives of girls and women were meant to have been bound to men regardless of the quality of the man or the consequences for the woman. The concept of women's freedom to choose their futures seems to have little place in such a world. Simply stated, Indian girls and women are taught from childhood to serve their husbands as if he is a deity (Bhattacharya 2000).

Conservative Hindus believe that the *Manusmriti* is divine, the words of Brahma. Contemporary feminist scholars, however, treat the *Manusmriti* as a set of precepts that create and justify the subordination of women. Both sides agree that the code points to the image of women as submissive and subordinate and that in everyday relationships, women should be docile and meek.

After the formation of the caste system, women in ancient India were singularly defined in terms of productivity in physical labor and as sexual beings, and they required domination. Caste rules reinforced women's subordination, and the merging of religious beliefs with material political and economic structures reduced women's place in society and allowed everyday life to devolve any thought or possibility of gender equity. Rules and practices of child marriage, prohibition of widow remarriage, the emergence of sati, and the barring of women from important religious rituals forced women to the margins of their own families and communities. Religious precepts further taught that women were inherently magical and capable of evil. As a class, women were unholy and could only gain *karma* through worship of their husbands (Dutta 2003).

Again, there was still variation in women's status and in gendered relationships in various regions of the subcontinent. Sati was not universally practiced, and caste differences allowed different outcomes for the everyday lives of widows. Lower castes, for example, tended toward greater tolerance of widow remarriage than did the upper castes. In royal families, wives were often the 'powers behind the throne'. Yet women were rarely if ever seated on the throne or allowed to become priests, sit on local panchayats, or become heads of households.

As Umar (1998) states, women in the *Manusmriti* are both the embodiment of purity and spiritual power as well as weak and dependent figures requiring continuous protection from men. In exchange for that protection, women are expected to use their powers in service of men.

The beliefs that women are magical have continued to the present day, albeit in varying degrees of literalness. For some, the historical beliefs of female magic persist as traditional superstitions or auspiciousness, while for others, the practice has continued only as a cultural expression of taste or expectation. For example, married Hindu women often put a streak of red vermillion in the part of their hair. For some women, this is merely an indication of marriage similar to the Western practice of wearing a wedding ring on the left-hand's fourth finger. For others, however, it is an act that has the power to keep their husbands safe and sound. Another example is wearing a toe ring. For some women, it is a style of adornment or indicator of marriage, but for others the ring protects their husbands' health.

Women's cosmological position in Hindu culture is that of magical, yet unholy persons whose spiritual powers should protect their husbands and ensure that the men in their lives outlive them. One of the ideological dictums that is used to justify the discrimination against widows that is found in many parts of India is that these women failed to shield their husbands from death.

The belief in the magical features or powers of women can have horrible consequences. The image of women as witches still haunts the Indian mind. In reporting on a murder case in the summer of 2016 in which a young man brutally axed his aunt to death believing she was a witch who cursed him with a disease, *India Today* cited government statistics that show that between 2001 and 2014 over 2,400 people, mostly poor women, were murdered for allegedly practicing witchcraft (Srivastava 2016). Women are highly vulnerable to charges of possessing evil powers.

Although beautiful women are extremely prized, superstitions lead many people to be suspicious of them. Women's allure is a tempting concession of the flesh that causes lustful desires and evil thoughts and can lead men to acts of sin. She may be beautiful on the outside, but on the inside, she is a temptress, an evil creature seeking to create spiritual havoc for men and trap them unawares. There seems to be no end to these superstitions, and women continue to be the victims.

## Are Girls Wanted?

There's an old sociology teaching game that asks this question: If a Martian[5] came to Earth, what would he see? The idea of the game was to teach students how to observe social behavior as objectively as possible, without any prior knowledge of the behavior or any personal investment or involvement in it. The game, at least as I always heard, assumed that a visiting Martian would be a male. Let us modernize this heuristic technique: What if the Martians were both male and female? Would a male Martian and a female Martian see Earth behavior differently? My guess is that they would, especially if they landed in India where they would see families taking extraordinary steps to avoid having daughters. Would the male Martian see son preference, female feticide, and violence against women as indications of something wrong or threatening about females, thus the need to limit them in number and control them in order to keep the peace? Would the female Martian, to the contrary, see these same phenomena as an atrocity?

One wonders if girls are wanted in many or even most Indian families. Son preference is a common, if not a staple, principle throughout the country. What is son preference about? Why do parents award such preference to sons over daughters? An abundance of studies have been conducted on the partiality given to sons over daughters and have uncovered numerous predictors of son preference, though the causes are varied. We can summarize these factors into three categories: economic, kinship, and religious.

Many champion an economic explanation of son preference. Wedding expenses are largely borne by the bride's family, and although illegal, the bride's family often contributes a dowry to enhance the new couple's welfare. Dowry prices have inflated dramatically over the last several decades and can be very high, sometimes forcing parents to liquidate their assets or be driven into indebtedness. One study conducted in Karnataka found that dowry prices average six times the annual income of the bride's family (Bloch, Rao, and Desai 2004). Among traditionalists, marriages remain arranged by the families. The so-called 'love marriages', however, usually are completed without dowry, but are disfavored by traditional families. Either way, the cost of the wedding remains high, largely, if not exclusively, borne by the bride's family and is a disincentive to having daughters, especially among families of low income and wealth, which is most of India.

Parenthetically, it is relevant to state that the alternative, an unmarried daughter, is a point of social shame and embarrassment in addition to the risk of having to support a daughter through adulthood. It is unthinkable, even scandalous, for a woman, or a man for that matter, not to marry by the age of 25 or so. Marrying off daughters, which is also considered a religious virtue, is considered a duty and obligation of parents (Stone and James 1995). Perhaps more importantly, offering one's daughter's chastity to another family is an act of honor, enhancing the bride's family's prestige within the village or caste (Basu 1999).

In addition to wedding and dowry costs, a second economic explanation for son preference is the need for son's labor. Given the poverty of many Indians, sons' labor is needed to support the family. Especially for poor rural families, more children result in more labor and enhanced family income, and sons generally produce more than girls.

Relatedly, since boys have greater access to education and are awarded substantially more economic opportunities than girls, men have a higher likelihood of 'hitting it rich', allowing the parents of the successful son to look forward to better economic support in old age. India does not have a formal, government-based social welfare program for the elderly, such as Social Security in the United States, or other retirement investment plans, which forces parents to rely upon their children for maintenance when they can no longer work and support themselves. In addition, for farmers, having a son protects family land, guaranteeing that their land will not be sold upon their death, which would happen if they only had daughters as survivors.

The reasons for son preference also seems to vary by gender. As Robitaille (2013) found, women prefer sons to daughters for economic reasons. Given that women, especially rural women, are more dependent upon men for their economic well-being, sons provide some insurance of support in the event their husbands pass away or become too frail to work. While economic opportunities are important to men for having sons, men are more likely to prefer sons for nonfinancial reasons. Robitaille's study showed that men also desire sons for religious reasons, to maintain the family name and prestige, and for consistency with their patriarchal principles, particularly their values about females.

A second set of factors thought to cause son preference is kinship systems that determine marriage patterns and the rules of gender roles within families. The idea here is that cultural norms dictate that sons support their elderly parents and that daughters will later contribute to the support of their husbands' parents, a system that presents as somewhat of an old-age emergency for parents of daughters. Having only daughters is a frightful situation that leads to parents worrying about how they will live during their senior years.

Relatedly other studies point to Indian kinship systems that position daughters to have little standing in their families of origin once they are married, thus becoming normatively and economically lost to parents, as the source of son preference. Traditional Indian families are patrilocal; daughters leave their families of origin to live with and among their in-laws. Their lives' focus becomes centered on their husband's family, which receives the benefit of a daughter-in-law's domestic and paid labor. In more traditional families, a daughter's parents receive little if any economic advantages of her adult work. Further, when parents stop working, cultural rules lead them to live with their sons, not their daughters. Even in cases where a daughter may be the 'favorite' child, living with her is not an option for respectable retirees. In many cultures of India, it is inauspicious for married daughters to present gifts or provide financial support to their birth families (Das Gupta 1987).

Another explanation for son preference is rooted in religion. Among Hindus, sons are needed to perform mandatory last rites rituals for parents. To bring salvation to the deceased, the *karta*, usually the eldest son, performs a set of rituals that prepares the soul for its departure to heaven. The *karta* circles the body three times, walking counter-clockwise so that the deceased is always on the left, and as prayers are recited to call the fire god Kravyada to burn the flesh and purify the soul, the *karta* lights the fire that consumes the body and releases the soul so that it can be reborn in its eternal continuance. The *karta* then assumes responsibility for his parent's ashes, preferably immersing them in the holy waters of the River Ganga. For believers, this ritual is critical. Without it, the soul wanders and cannot find its correct place.

Why must the eldest son, or other senior male relative in the absence of a son, serves as *karta*? Except among the most modern of Hindus, why are women generally excluded from performing this sacred task? A material explanation, as some have posited, would suggest that the practice began many centuries ago because men were more likely to possess the strength and endurance to create the friction necessary to start a fresh fire. Over time, greater religious significance was given to lighting the pyre, and ideologies were created to maintain and justify the funereal division of labor.

Others have said that women were prohibited from igniting the pyre because they were too emotionally frail to perform the *karta* duties without crying or losing their composure. Lighting the pyre required (and still does) emotional fortitude, which, according to this view, only men were believed to possess. As funeral teardrops are considered impure in the Hindu cosmology and that women were believed more likely to have an emotional response to lighting the pyre, people feared that women's lack of strength would lead to tears dripping upon the deceased, tainting its soul forever.

Another religion-based explanation is material and further gendered. It is possible that lighting the pyre, especially for one's father, is a ritual of social and material inheritance, a changing of the guard, if you will. Upon the death of the father, the eldest son becomes the head of the family and is entitled to the eldest's share of the inheritance, which is often more or better than the share his siblings receive. Lighting the pyre symbolically signified that the son was ready to assume his father's responsibilities in matters of family, business, and community.

There is an element (or possibility) of veracity in all three explanations. The primary significance of all of them is that they exclude women from participation, and since the successful release of the soul is absolutely necessary for the soul to be reborn in another earthly form (or to permit *moksha*, the freedom from *samsara*), traditional and religious Hindus fear not having a son to perform the rite.

In actuality, all of these conditions, economic, kinship, and religion, are relevant in son preference, and the answer to explaining why sons are preferred throughout the country and across caste and regional lines is in summing these variables together. The common denominator is that son preference is a product of the constructed assessment of the comparative worth of males and females. The two sexes are separated by value. It is an arbitrary sociocultural decision as to which family pays for a wedding or to whom dowry is given. We see this variation in a research finding that shows that gains in education correlate with lessened son preference (Pande and Astone 2007), and that son preference is stronger among higher caste groups since more property is at stake and strict rules are needed to perpetuate a family's wealth (Houska 1981). These findings indicate that son preference is a fluid concept, moving across time and place, forever shifting, as social conditions require.

Power, therefore, is the core value that shapes the desire for sons. Whether it is dividing wealth, maintaining systems that create laws and opportunities that favor men, or participating in significant religious rituals, the value of women in the Indian zeitgeist is muted in reference to men of similar caste. A high caste woman may hold high esteem among low caste villagers, but compared to high caste men, she is typically relegated to a relatively subordinate social position. The social construction of gender, therefore, is a process dating to ancient times when men seized command of their families, clans, and villages. What we see today is the continuation, the momentum of that primitive process in which an ideology or belief system is created to justify the division of wealth, power, and privilege, and that ideology is the social construction of gender.

*Dowry:* Although declared illegal in 1961 by the Dowry Prohibition Act and seemingly destined to become a historical artifact in the face of modernization and women's expanding role in the nation's market economy, dowry has not only persisted, but also appears to be increasing in both prevalence and value (Srinivasan and Lee 2004). Dowry is property transfer from the bride's family to the bridegroom's and can consist of personal items such as clothing and jewelry for the bride, household appliances such as a refrigerator, vehicles, tuition for the groom's education, and money. Originally a symbolic exchange of gifts and support for the new family, dowry soon became a pre-mortem inheritance to daughters because in many areas of north India, where dowry is believed to have originated, women could not inherit land and other tangible property, and compensation to the groom and his family were needed for supporting their daughter, given that women had little participation in the market economy (Srinivasan and Lee 2004).

Dowry, however, is more complicated than simple gift giving or avoiding inheritance for women. It is also a status marker for grooms, whose families, while arranging their marriage, seek to marry their sons to high caste and prestigious families. For brides, it is an opportunity for marrying into a higher caste or a better economic situation. The more dowry her family will offer, the greater the bargaining power they have to marry their daughter into a better lifestyle, which, in turn, could improve the parents' lot later on. Higher dowry can also act as a kind of insurance policy, helping protect daughters from overwork or violence in their husbands' households, over which brides' parents have little control.

With the rise of materialism and consumerism, dowry has evolved into demands for cash and modern consumer goods. With the economic fluctuations that accompany a capitalist economic system, which India has embraced in recent decades, financial stress of a Western sort has hit Indian families and individuals. Paired with gender inequality and patriarchy, the course of contemporary dowry practices is ripe for abusive acts.

Therefore, the potential for dowry extortion is high. Grooms and their families have been known to continue pushing the bride's family for more money or goods not only during the marriage negotiation process, but also well into the marriage after the wedding. On many occasions, this psychological and social pressure turns violent, causing India to create a new crime statistic – dowry death. Dowry death, sometimes known as 'bride burning', has become a serious public health issue in India. It is an interesting statistical category in that it includes both homicide and suicide; the common thread is that a woman's death, whether self-inflicted or willingly caused by others, is fueled by the pressures, harassment, and physical violence related to demands for money or wealth from her family. As stated in the Indian Penal Code, dowry death occurs:

> When the death of a woman is caused by any burns or other bodily injury, or occurs other than under normal circumstances, within seven years of her marriage, and it is shown that soon before her death she was subjected to cruelty or harassment by her husband or by any relative of her husband's for, or in connection with any demand for dowry. (cited in Kumar 2003)

According to national statistics from the Ministry of Home Affairs (2010, 2013), there were over 6,000 officially recognized dowry deaths in 1997, and the count has increased since then. Table 2.1 shows the number of dowry deaths recorded by the National Crime Records Bureau from 2011 to 2014. It is important to remember that these are official counts representing only reported and recorded cases. As shall be seen in Chapter 3, official registers are quite likely understating the actual incidence of this crime. The key issue here is that this is a crime that happens with alarming frequency: officially roughly 24 times each day, once an hour (*Times of India* 2013).

**Table 2.1**

*'Dowry deaths' from 2011 to 2014*

| *Year* | *Dowry Deaths* |
|---|---|
| 2011 | 8,618 |
| 2012 | 8,233 |
| 2013 | 8,083 |
| 2014 | 8,650 |

It is common for Westerners to see dowry deaths as a feature or natural outcropping of traditional Hindu and Asian cultures. Such an approach, however, is insufficient and misleading. Violence against women is not conceptualized as a cultural phenomenon in the United States or in Europe, then why should that proposition have validity in India?

As Narayan (1997) and Rudd (2001) rightly contend, cultural explanations of dowry deaths neglect the depth of patriarchal norms and the structure of social control mechanisms that target women as a social class. A cultural perspective of such violence does not allow us to comprehend the 'otherness' of women in everyday Indian life and to recognize the recentness of dowry murders (Narayan 1997).

## Conclusion

In all cultures, when a baby is born, two questions are asked immediately: is the baby healthy and is it a boy or a girl. These questions immediately address and define the infant in terms of its body and the meanings of that body as 'abled' and gendered. Babies' lives, without knowledge of their talents, propensities, or temperaments, are now and forever organized by social forces that provide opportunities to act, learn, work, and simply pursue life. The social construction of gender has real consequences for men and women, creating different life pathways and chances for varying forms of joy and pain.

The essentialization of women reduces the capability of their bodies to bearers of children, preferably sons, and sexual and material labor sources for men. The female body, in many segments of Indian society, seems to have little other ability, a dynamic that creates a disproportionately high physical burden on the body in the forms of violence and, as shall be seen, the meaning of the consequences of violence. Domestic and sexual violence occurs to women because of the definitions of femaleness held by the perpetrator of the violence and the sociocultural environment that foments and reinforces those definitions. Where women are essentialized and reduced to minimal expectations, violence against them is more likely, and oddly enough, women are often blamed for the violence they endure. As women are reduced to the barest, essential nature, there is little tolerance for exception, and the social climate around them will use all measures available to punish women who attempt to exercise their agency.

Despite the seemingly gloomy image of women's well-being in India, we must avoid thinking that Indian girls and women are downtrodden and emotionless beings eking out a living in a subservient and beaten-down existence. Throughout history, girls and women indeed did and still do have lives of joy, play, and laughter that coexist with the pain and suffering of living in the patriarchal world that marginalizes them (Lal 2013). Despite their constrained and somewhat incarcerated milieu, the struggle against marginality in everyday life is not soul-less; girls and women know playfulness and have their own sources of happiness and delight (Lal 2013). As will be shown later on, women suffering some of the starkest social degradations respond with great resolve and determination. The female spirit is strong in India and is not easily defeated.

## Notes

1. I encourage readers to refer to Alison Stone's book for an excellent review of essentialism.
2. As Bourdieu argued, such conventions are a consequence of inter-elite competition, rather than based on what is functional to reach social goals, productivity, or well-being. See Paula England (2016).
3. I offer apologies to historians who have worked for decades to understand the transformation of Vedic India. There are many excellent histories on Vedic India and the formation of the caste system. A comprehensive historical analysis is beyond the scope of the present study.
4. For example, one theory suggests that in early farming societies, women used simple hoes to tend to agricultural plots and worked alongside men in the fields. The invention of the animal-powered plow made the hoe, and therefore women, redundant. In turn, women became economically expendable, despite their other economic productivity, and consequently, subordinate.
5. When I first learned this game, intelligent and civilized though warlike, life on Mars was still the stuff of science fiction. Visiting Martians were always male.

# 3

# Burning Women

## Facts and Treatments

> If my daughter or sister engaged in pre-marital activities and disgraced herself and allowed herself to lose face and character by doing such things, I would most certainly take this sort of sister or daughter to my farmhouse, and in front of my family, I would put petrol on her and set her alight.
>
> —A.P. Singh, attorney,
> interviewed in *India's Daughter: The Life of Jyoti Singh* 2012

India is a land like no other. Often perceived as an impoverished but peaceful place guided by Gandhi's principles of nonviolence, outsiders often think of Indians as vegetarian and practitioners of yoga who spend their lives in ashrams alongside contemplative swamis meditating on the mysteries of their exotic religion. The stereotyped image of the 'docile Hindu' has pervaded the subcontinent since early colonial times. The British not only judged Hindus to be industrious, but also contented and obedient, and according to most colonials were a cheerful and deferential lot who made ideal subjects of the empire. Perhaps what led the British to these conclusions, as some have said, was the interpretation of eight centuries of Muslim dominance of Hindu India, Hindus' obedience to strict social roles associated with caste, and the belief in the inevitability of fate as a genetic disposition towards submissiveness and compliance to authority. This stereotype has persisted to contemporary times and has helped conceal a society rife with both communal and domestic violence, not only among Hindus, but among India's other religious groups as well.

Thus, India is no timid society. Violence or the risk of violence is substantial at all levels of society. At the institutional level, India is a militarized state that boasts of a nuclear arsenal and huge military forces, the latter having been called to action many times since independence. And, as a side note, prior to independence, a majority of soldiers in the Royal Army of India were Indian, not British, which indicates a certain comfort with police and military jobs. At the social group level, sectarian violence has become a stain on the image of India as the world's largest democracy. Mob violence takes many forms: neighborhoods are burned to the ground, children are killed with swords and machetes, Dalit men are lynched, and women are raped to discredit them in their own communities. These events occur with alarming frequency for a state that prides itself on maintaining a unified national identity despite great religious and cultural diversity.

Interpersonally, domestic violence is epidemic in the subcontinent. As shall be seen, research indicates that one-third of married women report having been the victim of violence from their husbands, and much of this violence is maiming or fatal. Countless numbers of girls and women have been slapped, hit, punched, or worse by the men in their lives.

Lastly, suicide rates in India are higher than many think they should be. Suicide, especially when committed by women, is often a tragic consequence of the violence that occurs in other corners of society, particularly violence at home, as we shall see later in this chapter.

One of the most sinister forms of violence against people in India is burning, a crime that particularly targets women.

Dousing a woman with kerosene and then tossing a lighted match on her, or throwing acid on her face and torso, are not uncommon forms of violence in India. Kerosene, used widely as cooking fuel in Indian kitchens, and acid, which is found easily throughout India, are weapons capable of terrible consequences. Survivors of such attacks are scarred permanently, and many lose the use of all or parts of their faces, arms, or hands. Whereas a kerosene fire often leaves a person with charred-looking flesh and keloid welts that are unsightly and painful, acid often renders skin looking like burned, sagging, discolored wax, and because fire and acid can burn off body parts, it is common to find victims without lips, eyelids, or fingers.

In addition to the physical effects of being burned, the psychosocial consequences of both the attack and the subsequent scars can cause additional and sometimes more severe distress and pain. Disfigurement, for any reason and to any degree, typically has a negative valence; that is, people frequently perceive disfigurement as implying that something is desperately wrong with the disfigured person.

The goal of this chapter is to present the social context of burning women, which includes the 'bride burning' crime discussed in the previous chapter. The present chapter will discuss incidence and prevalence, risk factors, and a social profile of victims. In addition, a short review of medical treatments for severely disfigured burn victims will be presented.

## How Men Burn Women

> Police in Jharkhand state arrested the husband and parents-in-law of a young woman for allegedly burning her and her baby girl alive. The primary motive is suspected to be dowry-related, as alleged by the parents of Annu Devi, 22, who died from severe burn wounds in a hospital three days after the attack. The one

year-old baby died instantly. Three suspects were arrested. (CNN, 3 February 2014)

The cultures of the Indian subcontinent have an ancient history of burning women. The best-known example is sati. Banned by British colonials in 1829 as a hideous and savage ritual, the sati is the ceremonial practice in which a widow throws herself on her husband's funeral pyre in order to join him in death. A sati, which is the title bestowed on the participating widow, becomes a woman of honor and a point of pride for her family (Datta 1988). In Halvad, a small town in the Indian state of Gujarat, there is a historic sati site where widows of fallen Rajput warriors of the 17th and 18th centuries first made clay imprints of one arm, bent at a 90-degree angle, before throwing themselves onto the flames consuming their husbands' remains. Despite their age, the impressions on these monuments are exact in their detail. The lines of the satis' hands are particularly eerie; the bangles on the wrists and rings on fingers still show the artistry of their crafting. Scores of these *paliyas* dot this site, which, while considered a sacred place among Hindus, is puzzling and somewhat emotionally taxing to Western visitors.

Sati was not practiced throughout India. In regions such as Rajasthan, Gujarat, and Bengal, among others, sati was common and widely accepted, but in other parts of the country sati was either not expected or unknown. Although rare in contemporary times, sati lingers within the Indian consciousness, and the country still has 250 sati temples. Various media reports estimate the number of satis since independence to be between 40 and 60. On some occasions, reports of a widow committing sati reveal more malevolent situations, such as in the highly publicized sati of Roop Kanwar (Sen 2001), an 18-year-old woman widowed in 1987. After the sati, questions were raised as to whether Roop

Kanwar's sati was voluntary or the result of intense social pressure and coercion to commit the act. Many family members and villagers were later charged with drugging the young bride and forcing her onto the pyre, although all defendants eventually were cleared of wrongdoing. Whether voluntary or pushed into sati, Roop Kanwar died because of a belief that women should end their lives upon their husband's death.

The origins of sati are unclear, though the rite has long had both sacred and secular meaning. Many conservative Hindus believe that sati enhances their late husband's spiritual salvation. Sacrificing herself for her husband's redemption is the highest expression of a woman's devotion and is rewarded by revering the sati as a goddess (Harlan 1994: 80). The historic belief is that women are magical beings whose lot in life is to use their powers to ensure that their husbands outlive them. When a husband dies before his wife, she is judged to have failed in her sacred duty, bringing dishonor upon her family.

In a more sociological light, sati is seen as a function of broad gender inequality in which women's lives are cheap unless in the service of fathers and husbands. Widowhood has long been an undesirable status in most India communities. Treated as outcasts, widows were essentially subtracted from social life: they were secluded and expected to keep their heads covered and sometimes shaved; they were the last in households to eat and were usually required to eat alone; and they were rarely invited to social functions. Belief in the religious meanings of sati, the weight of the family and personal shame, and the knowledge that life as a widow could be difficult, if not cruel, drove widows to self-immolation. Life for Indian widows is only somewhat better today, as widowhood is still stigmatized in many areas (Agarwal 1998; Nussbaum 2000).

In present times, ritualistic woman burning is illegal and morally contemptible to the vast majority of Indians. The case of a 60-year-old Rajasthani widow illustrates the point. Upon the death of her husband in 2009, Sharbati Bai, seeing life as a widow as too difficult to face, attempted to join her deceased husband on the pyre that would consume his body. She was restrained by villagers and the police, however, and was saved from a horrible death (*Times of India* 2009).

Indeed sati is on the cusp of becoming a relic of history; however, the sentiments behind sati linger in the Indian psyche, and men's behavior toward women in general is only slightly better than in times past. Nonetheless, burning remains as a means to discard or punish women who are unwanted or 'wrong acting', and compels us to consider Linda Hess' hypothesis: 'Would it be an unfair stretch to associate (Sita's image in the sati pyre) with the brideburning incidents that have been increasing in north India in the last thirty years?' (1999: 23). Although change toward the recognition of women's rights is slowly developing, India remains rooted in deep-seated patriarchal values that perpetuate gender relationships best described as feudalistic. Women's lives in India are laborious and measured largely by beauty and the number of sons they produce.

## Acid and Kerosene Burns

Unlike sati, contemporary burn violence against women is more likely to occur in a private, rather than a public arena, and is more geographically widespread throughout the subcontinent than sati ever was. If official state records were used to estimate the frequency of burn assaults, however, it would be easy to conclude that its incidence is quite low, if not rare, as the crime is not often reported to police and is seldom prosecuted. Few perpetrators are punished. Research, in comparison to official reports, paints a more alarming picture of how often the crime occurs in South Asia.

Rates of incidence of the two forms are difficult to determine since police and hospital reports do not necessarily specify how burn victims are injured. Although the present study focuses on women burned with kerosene, which occurs more frequently than acid burns, a quick review of the differences between the types of violence is in order because they operate somewhat differently in terms of social dynamics and medical consequences.

Both acid and kerosene are commonly found throughout India, and the ease with which the materials involved in burning are obtained facilitates the high incidence of burning as a suicide method, weapon for attack, and source of accidents. Sulfuric, nitric, hydrochloric, tannic, and formic acids are commonplace and found in the countless jewelry shops and auto repair businesses located throughout the country (Shahidul, Choudhary, and Mahmud 2001). Acids are also used in the huge cloth dyeing and tanning industries and, unlike in Western households, are found in homes as a product for cleaning bathrooms and kitchens.

Kerosene, a liquid hydrocarbon fuel, is similarly accessible in Indian homes and used as a cheap cooking fuel. Kerosene stoves and containers are ubiquitous, especially among poorer families, which of course, constitute much of the Indian population. Kerosene is highly combustible and accounts for thousands of accidental household fires. That accidental kerosene fires are common is one reason it is used as a weapon in domestic violence and accounts for why burn attacks are usually carried out in private social spaces, especially in homes where they can be explained away as accidents.

Although the incidence and prevalence of burn assaults are imprecise, the details of burn attacks are well-known. The attacks usually are carried out in private social spaces where the perpetrator tosses the acid or kerosene (obviously a lit match is required as well) onto the victims. Cases where acid has been shot through a syringe have also been documented. If the perpetrator and victim are not married, acid burns may occur in public places, which allow the attacker to speedily disappear into the mass of humanity that is India. A 'drive-by' acid toss by someone on a motorcycle, for example, maximizes the likelihood of escape and makes identifying the attacker difficult. Another common method is flinging acid through windows while a victim is studying or sleeping.

The consequences of these attacks are unbelievably harsh. The pain incurred by being burned is long and unimaginable and is among the most severe types of pain people can experience. Victims wail in tortuous agony, the excruciating pain escalating as the acid or fire spreads further and deeper into victims' bodies. Although chemical and thermal (fire) burns have similar effects in terms of the damage they cause, they have different sensations at the onset of contact. Acid feels like water when it first hits the skin, wet with no immediate burning sensation. In only a few seconds, however, a searing feeling begins, rising in intensity until the acid is washed away or neutralized (Shahidul et al. 2001). The pain of thermal burns, victims report, is more immediate. Fire not only damages skin, but also penetrates to the muscles, bones, nerves, and blood vessels, inflicting deep body pain and injury.

Acid and kerosene fire can burn away functional parts of the head (ears, lips, and eyes) and parts of arms (fingers), as well as skin, leaving victims horribly disfigured and impaired. Victims who lose their eyelids, for instance, have permanent unnatural facial expressions and are unable to blink. The inability to blink causes eyes to become unbearably dry and covered with dust and other particles. Ears and noses burn off rather easily as do lips, fingers, and muscles, tendons, and ligaments. Burns can cause deeper internal damage too. Some acids such as tannic and formic are absorbed quickly by the skin and can produce systemic harm such as renal failure (Shahidul and Mahmud 2001) and fire by kerosene also can affect breathing as inhaled smoke obstructs airways. All in all, acid and thermal burns create among the most debilitating injuries imaginable. In less than a minute, a person can become a charred hulk of skin, blackened and dismembered and immediately unrestorably ugly in the eyes of most people around them.

## Incidence and Prevalence

As mentioned earlier, prevalence and incidence are tough to determine; however, analysts and scholars agree that the overall incidence of burns implies that they pose a significant public health problem in the subcontinent. The World Health Organization (2016) estimates that more than 1 million people are moderately or severely burned every year in India. Girls and women endure more burns than boys and men because they have greater exposure to risk, which is a function of the commonness of open fire cooking and unsafe stoves. High mortality among young married women due to burns has become especially disturbing (Sanghavi, Bhalla, and Das 2009). In fact, in 1998, burns ranked among the top 15 causes of death in India, giving the country a unique distinction in the modern world as the only country to have burns rank in the top causes of death (Batra 2003). Indian hospitals treat over a half million women for burns each year (Jaiswal et al. 2007). Studies estimate that nationally girls and women account for

65 per cent of burn deaths, and burns explain one-fourth of all female mortality (Sanghavi et al. 2009).

Regional studies show similar but varying results. For example, a study of a rural health district on Maharashtra found that 23 per cent of all deaths between 1997 and 2001 were attributed to burns; over 80 per cent of those cases were girls and women (Batra 2003). Roughly half the cases were ruled suicidal, 2 per cent were officially recorded as homicide, and the remaining half were accidents. A study of 328 consecutive forensic autopsies of women aged 12–49 in Mangalore found that 93.6 per cent were unnatural deaths, as would be expected for bodies assigned to forensic study (Padubidri et al. 2013). Of these, the top three causes of death were burns, poison, and hanging, which accounted for 69.5 per cent of the deaths. Just over 45 per cent were ruled suicides, and 43.6 per cent were declared accidents. Homicides accounted for 4.6 per cent of the cases, as legally defined. All of the homicides were married women, and a third of them were burn victims.

One study, however, found slightly different but important findings. In a five-year study conducted between 2008 and 2012 in Lucknow, Kumar and his associates (2013) discovered that 60 per cent of all deaths assigned to autopsy were attributed to burns. Of the flame deaths, about 38 per cent were ruled suicide and 37 per cent were deemed accidental. Of significance, however, 24.1 per cent of the burn deaths were considered homicides, a marked difference from other reports and official statistics.

Consequently, the actual extent of the crime is not known, but most agree that the number of accidents reported by hospitals and police departments is overstated and the number of assaults is understated; that is, crimes against women are grossly underreported. Official police records do not produce results comparable to those of women's advocacy groups and the many researchers who claim that official reports exaggerate the incidence of accidents in order to conceal or disguise domestic violence and homicide (Sanghavi et al. 2009; Sawhney 1989; Sharma, Harish, Sharma, and Vij 2002). What is often mistaken or falsely recorded as an accident is in fact an attempted homicide packaged with deniability and a legal defense. What is more, suicides by Indian women are commonly a sad conclusion to severe and persistent domestic violence. It is a tragic end to a life of misery and torture.

Of course the main question regarding these assaults is why they happen. While it is clear that the act of attacking a woman with acid or fire has the single purpose of inflicting pain, physical damage, or death (Peck 2012), research has not identified a single causal factor that explains burn attacks (Umar 1998). Nonetheless, a number of factors has been recognized as causal conditions, suggesting multiple pathways to this form of violence. Among unmarried female victims, most are attacked after rejecting a sexual advance or marriage proposal. Married victims, on the other hand, are subject to dowry violence in which the husband, or on some occasions an in-law, attempts to extort more dowry from the victim's family. Although dowry is frequently named as the cause of burning wives and is often considered synonymous with bride burning in popular media and discussions (Belur et al. 2014; Kumar and Tripathi 2004), research has yet to determine how frequently such crimes are committed. Kumar's studies have found that only 5 per cent of burn assaults are connected to dowry problems (Kumar et al. 2013; Kumar et al. 2014); however, others, such as Shaha and Mohanty (2006) report that about 55 per cent of burns-related deaths are due to homicide and that half of those are a consequence of dowry quarrels.

Oftentimes women are burned because their husbands want to punish them for some real or imagined transgression or simply to get rid of them in order to marry someone else. Rigid divorce laws and a strong social stigma against divorced individuals force many into desperation (Umar 1998), making violence against oneself or a spouse preferable to civil separation. For men, being a widower is a more sympathetic figure than a man who is divorced, thereby increasing the odds that he will remarry and maybe gain a second dowry.

These murders and attempted murders are frequently disguised as accidents or suicides as family members and the police are not always straightforward in presenting accounts of the burns (Belur et al. 2014). Good police and medical forensic practices, however, can often distinguish accidents from attacks. For example, law enforcement can identify concealed intentional violence by detecting kerosene odors that would not exist in an accidental fire and the pre-morbid removal of jewelry, which would be unlikely in an accident. Homicide cases may also be recognized by delays in seeking treatment and failure to notify the wife's family of the 'accident'. Also, in a truly accidental fire, nearby in-laws or other family members and neighbors usually present with injuries sustained while attempting to put out the fire (Peck 2012). In an act of deliberate violence, others are not usually hurt. Sometimes witness accounts do not match in cases of homicide, and if the woman survives, her description of the attack may differ from others. Further, survivors of actual attacks are often more reluctant to talk in front of in-laws than true accident victims (Peck 2012). Policing the police is often effective in these cases as officers are occasionally bribed to report a fire incidence as accidental. (It should be noted that men are also targets of this kind of violence, albeit far less frequently. Women are six times more likely than men to be burned to death, including by accident (Kumar et al. 2014). Men who are intentionally burned are more likely to be attacked as a result of property disputes, arguments with other men, or business competition.)

## Profile of Burned Women

Despite the lack of reliability in determining incidence, many studies have attempted to create a profile of burned women. These reports are limited in scope because they have used samples limited to a particular hospital or police jurisdiction. Still, from these studies we can identify several key patterns in victims' social characteristics. Women in lower social class positions risk increasingly higher exposure to burn attack than higher status women (Belur et al. 2014; Kumar et al. 2014), which corresponds with findings that victims are disproportionately poorly educated or are illiterate (Belur et al 2014; Shaha and Mohanty 2006; Sharma et al. 2014). Victims are more common in rural areas, almost exclusively Hindu in religion (Shaha and Mohanty 2006; Stone and James 1995), and in childbearing ages (18–40) (Kumar et al. 2013; Shaha and Mohanty 2006). Victims were also attacked primarily at home and in the daytime (Shaha and Mohanty 2006). Further research by Kumar and associates (2014) found that women who are burned to death are likely to have experienced two or more stressful events, such as economic distress, relationship problems, and marital conflicts, compared to women not burned by husbands. These problems, especially marital strife, suggest that burn attacks are not often one-off events of conflict, but rather are embedded in a web of marital discord and perhaps other violence at the hands of their husbands or other family members.

Most research on burn deaths relies upon autopsy data, thus the studies have neither complete nor sufficient information to create an in-depth sociological profile of women victims. Other research only reviews the most extreme cases such as when a woman has died from burns or has received prolonged hospitalization.

The Demographic and Health Surveys (DHS), however, provides means to describe the lives of women who survived burnings by their husbands. The DHS is a large-scale, national-level random sample of women that focuses primarily on women's reproductive and maternal health and is largely funded by the United States government through its USAID program, working with local governments around the world to collect data to inform national policy-makers and planners and researchers about the health of women and children. Data were last collected in India in 2006 (Demographic and Health Surveys (India) 2006a, 2006b).

In that year, the Indian panel began asking questions about domestic and intimate partner violence, having defined such violence as a women's health issue. Women were asked if they had ever been victims of violence, and if so, what kinds of violence they had experienced, who perpetrated that violence, and, to some extent, the degree of injury resulting from assaults. Respondents were also asked about emotional abuse and their husbands' attempts to control them in everyday life.

Of the 1,24,385 women in the total sample, 69,484 were selected randomly for questions about domestic violence. A further subset of 22,669 was asked about wounds that resulted from domestic violence. Of that latter subsample, 429 women (1.9%) reported having been severely burned by their husbands. Since the sample is randomly selected, we can extrapolate to the larger population the prevalence rate of such burns. Taking census data for 2006 and estimating the number of women 18 years of age and older as roughly 390 million, we would estimate a prevalence of over 50,00,000 women who have ever been burned by their husbands.[1] This is, sad to say, an alarmingly large number of women burned intentionally and maliciously by their spouses. Note that this figure, since it is based on randomly located survivors, projects the number of survivors and does not include those who died.

Using these data, we can get an image of burned women's social profile, compared to women in the sample who were not similarly attacked. A brief statistical detour is necessary to illustrate the poverty of well-being that these women endure and a glimpse into the lives they lead.

## Social Characteristics

As other studies have found, burn attacks appear in families throughout the country and in all levels of society. Yet, some women are more likely targets of this crime. Consistent with studies referenced earlier, women with less education and who are illiterate have higher rates of victimization, as Tables 3.1 and 3.2 show, when compared to the general population of women in India. Approximately three of four burned women have only primary education or less, compared to 46 per cent of women in general. Similarly literacy rates are far lower among burn victims; two-thirds of burn victims are illiterate compared to roughly 35 per cent of the general population.

**Table 3.1**
*Education*

| *Education* | *General Population* | *Burn Victims* |
|---|---|---|
| No Education | 32.0% | 56.6% |
| Incomplete Primary | 7.8% | 9.6% |
| Complete Primary | 6.5% | 8.4% |
| Incomplete Secondary | 37.2% | 21.4% |
| Complete secondary | 6.1% | 2.3% |
| Higher | 10.4% | 1.6% |

**Table 3.2**
*Literacy*

| | *General Population* | *Burned Victims* |
|---|---|---|
| Cannot Read at All | 35.5% | 63.6% |
| Minimal Reading Ability | 4.9% | 4.7% |
| Literate | 59.6% | 31.7% |

Education and literacy are risk factors for burn violence, and higher rates of both provide some degree of protection, suggesting that women with less human capital and self-empowerment are more vulnerable to gendered aggression of this type. Education provides a number of buffering factors such as heightened self-awareness and efficacy, increased avenues of social and economic support, and a lower likelihood of dependency. With fewer tangible options, women are more likely to become trapped in desperate situations and fall victim to men who have similarly poor social and economic skills. Since about 30 per cent of burn victims place in the top two quintiles of DHS' wealth index, compared to 55 per cent of the general population of women, it is clear that economic factors play a role in domestic burn violence. The burden of stress produced by poverty and near poverty is felt in families, as research has long demonstrated. The family is indeed not a 'haven in the heartless world' of contemporary society, but the locality of the stress and frustrations generated by inequality, consumerism, powerlessness, and the absence of health care and education services that are available to others.

### *Abuse of Women*

Sociology has long wrestled with theoretical explanations of linking macro social structures with micro, or everyday, behavior. Sometimes it helps merely to 'see' it, and one way to do that is to model the reach of the patriarchy, a macro-level social construct, into the everyday lives of women and men. By assessing the emotional climate and degree of male dominance in families, we can visualize the penetration of patriarchal intrusion into a family. The more that men control and abuse women, the safer it is to assume that the husbands have internalized the precepts of the patriarchal order.

There are several ways to detect patriarchal conditions in male–female relationships: Do men control their wives' behavior? Do men emotionally abuse their wives? Do men violently assault them? The DHS allows us this window into the patriarchy, and we can observe if gendered dominant relations have any role in women's likelihood of burn attacks.

*Control:* DHS operationalizes spouse control as an index score of six types of controlling behavior, as shown below. Women in the sample were asked to state whether or not their husbands had committed any of these acts.

1. Husband gets jealous if they talk with other men.
2. Husband accuses her of unfaithfulness.
3. Husband does not allow her to meet her girlfriends.
4. Husband limits contact with family.
5. Husband insists on knowing where she is.
6. Husband does not trust her with money.

The findings are stark. Among women in general, about 61 per cent reported having never experienced any of these controls on their behavior, and roughly 28 per cent stated that their husbands had committed one or two of these acts; only a little over 5 per cent reported four or more such experiences (Table 3.3).

Of the burn attack victims, however, the control of their behavior by their husbands was far more stringent. About 17 per cent reported at least one marital control, almost twice that of women in general, and 35.6 per cent stated that they had suffered four or more, ten times the rate of the non-burned women. Almost 13 per cent of burn victims recounted that they had experienced all six of the controlling abuse conditions, an astounding number compared to the general population (0.5%): They were 24 times more likely to suffer all six situations.

**Table 3.3**
*The number of control issues experienced*

| *Issues* | *Number of Control* *General Population* | *Burn Victims* |
|---|---|---|
| 0 | 61.0% | 18.9% |
| 1 | 15.8% | 17.0% |
| 2 | 12.2% | 15.4% |
| 3 | 5.6% | 13.1% |
| 4 | 2.9% | 12.1% |
| 5 | 1.4% | 10.7% |
| 6 | 0.5% | 12.8% |

Husbands who have burned and perhaps almost killed their wives are far more likely to try to control their partners' behavior by limiting their contact with others, restraining their geographic and financial freedom, and accusing them of betrayal. The consequence of such controlling behavior is to restrict women's ability to move about and exercise their own agency and will. Such behavior is typical of abusers and implies that violence is merely a part of an environment of control and intimidation.

Controlling women is an essential expression of patriarchy. Without an ideology that both instructs and reinforces such control, it is unlikely to occur. It is perhaps a human quality to control what we believe we own. Therefore to 'own' women is to control them. This signature of patriarchy betrays any pretense of the humanness of women. Instead, it points to women as an 'other' subject, ranked lower than men and subject to control and dominance by men.

*Violence and Abuse:* Many years ago Lenore Walker (1979) discovered that violent couples follow a pattern that she labeled the continuum of violence. This concept describes how abuse advances over time from relatively less harmful to severe. Offenders do not begin their abuse by hitting or kicking; these forms of violence are too severe for a new relationship to deal with. Rather, violent men begin with emotional abuse. They will humiliate or denigrate their partners, neglect their needs, follow them around, question them about their activities, and move to cut them off from their friends and relatives. Then abusers begin relatively light violence against their wives. They may push their partners against a wall, pull their hair, or hit them with an open hand. If they are not punished by the police and the courts or other family members or feel sufficiently guilty and remorseful to stop themselves from committing further violence, they will progress to more dangerous types of violence. Most offenders do not continue to lethal forms of violence, but eventually reach their own plateau of severity and do not go beyond it (Furr 1997: 363). The men who burn their wives have no such plateau or self-control or other agents of authority forcing them to stop. They follow the continuum to its unfortunate end.

*Emotional Violence:* As Walker's continuum of violence model predicts, intimate partner violence begins with emotional abuse. Although we cannot determine the sequence of abusive behavior of the abusers identified in the DHS data, we can show from these DHS data if burn victims experience emotional violence in the form of spousal humiliation, threats of harm, and insults to the point of causing hurt feelings. As with spousal control, emotional abuse befell burned women more frequently than women in general (see Table 3.4). Non-burned women suffered emotional abuse at a rate of about 14 per cent, whereas burned women were five times more likely to have experienced one of these insults to their integrity. Just fewer than 70 per cent of these women were subjected to emotional violence, and half of these episodes were recent, occurring within the last 12 months (these data are not shown in the table). The high incidence of emotional abuse among burned women indicates that physical violence does not happen in a vacuum. It is accompanied by other maltreatment.

**Table 3.4**

*Prevalence of emotional violence*

| | *Emotional* | |
|---|---|---|
| *Violence* | *General Population* | *Burn Victims* |
| Humiliation | 11.5% | 62.2% |
| Threaten with Harm | 5.0% | 6.6% |
| Insult | 7.3% | 50.3% |
| Any Occurrence | 14.1% | 69.7% |

*Web of Violence:* Moving onward with the continuum of violence guide, and as would be expected from the vast literature on intimate partner violence, a severe form of violence such as burning is expected to be partnered with other forms of direct physical violence. It is reasonable to assume that these women experience other types of violence prior to and perhaps after the burn.

As the continuum model submits, the usual pattern of violence in families is one of escalation in both physicality and consequences. It is unusual for men to initiate relatively severe violence without first experimenting with less physical means to see what level of abuse will be tolerated by his wife, family, and his own emotional and behavioral limits. What is likely is that before a man hits or shoves his wife, he begins with psychological and social abuse, such as humiliating and insulting her and controlling her contacts with friends and family. Men build their violent 'careers' over time, becoming increasingly ferocious. Before they hit with a weapon or attempt to kill, these men typically follow a progression of emotional abuse, then less dangerous slapping or pushing, before intensifying to violence that is more likely to cause injury and even death. In general, without intervention or personal change, men who hit their female partners will progress through the continuum. Where one sees severe violence, one should see lesser forms occurring first. If this model is true, a kerosene attack, a highly violent and aggressive act, is merely one part of the violence that ensnares the family, and is perhaps the most visible assault amid the countless humiliations and attacks these women have endured.

Women who are burned by their husbands live in a web of violence, just as the continuum of violence model predicts. The burn survivors have suffered violence in addition to the kerosene attacks, and in many cases the violence continues after their burns. Data from the DHS lead us to believe that burn victims must live a life of continuous fear and pain, never knowing what violence and insufferable shame awaits them. They are abused emotionally and controlled behaviorally, and they are beaten and sexually assaulted.

Table 3.5 reports that over half of burn victims suffer relatively less severe violence,[2] such as being punched, hit, or kicked, than women who do not suffer violent burns. Almost all burned women have been slapped, punched, or shaken violently. Compared to Indian women in general, burned women are eight times more likely to be kicked or hit with a fist than women in the general population, and are 15 times more likely to be attacked with a weapon. Not shown in the table is the finding that just over half of burn victims have been punched, hit, or kicked within the last year, and over one-third (68%) have been slapped in the last 12 months. The violence seems never-ending.

**Table 3.5**

*Incidence of Violence*

| | *General Population* | *Burn Victims* |
|---|---|---|
| Punched, Shook, or Something Thrown at Them | 12% | 86% |
| Slapped | 30% | 99% |
| Hit with a Fist or Something Harmful | 9% | 79% |
| Kicked or Dragged | 10% | 79% |
| Attacked with a Weapon | 2% | 29% |
| Sexual Violence | 8% | 50% |

The DHS further distinguishes between nonsexual violence and sexual assault (forced and unwanted sex). Sexual violence by spouses is common among burned women: husbands of half of the burn victims have forced unwanted sex on their wives. (Again, the violence is continuous: almost two-thirds of victims who have suffered forced, unwanted sex acts by their husbands have done so within the last 12 months.) About 80 per cent of women not burned by their husbands have been sexually abused by them, meaning that burn victims are more than six times more likely to be sexually assaulted than women in the general population.

The image of violence is made more complete when we add a couple of other statistical findings. First, burned women are also more likely to have been physically injured by their mothers-in-law (5.1% to 0.3%) and fathers-in-law (1.9% to 0.1%) than other women. Second, about 36 per cent of burned women saw their fathers beat their mothers compared to 16.7 per cent of the general population of women. Clearly violence has consumed the lives of burned women, leaving them scared, fearful, vulnerable, and lacking a safe harbor for escape.

What does this mean? As Hamby and Grych (2013: 107) state, 'No form of violence is an isolated phenomenon'. Women who are burned by their husbands live unsafe lives. The 'bride burning' is likely not a one-off event; rather, it is a step in the escalation of violence that ends in lethality. These women are controlled, abased, and abused, and all before they are burned, but we only hear about them if and when they become a subject for the media or another police or hospital statistic.

Given the amount of violence against Indian women that this study, as well many others, have revealed, all studies of Indian women and families should begin with Kumar and colleagues' statement: 'Domestic violence is a commonly accepted part of family life in India' (Kumar, Gupta, and Abraham 2002). At least one-third of married Indian women have experienced some form of intimate partner violence, and the police and the courts seem willing to let the offenses go unpunished. Prosecutions are few, and convictions are practically rarc. Wc must also rccognizc that wc should not focus only on burn attacks. We must look at the pervasiveness of violence because burns are not isolated, solitary violent events. We overstate their political and theoretical significance because the real issue is violence against women, not solely burn violence. If agents of social authority move to intervene sooner in intimate partner violence, it is likely that burn violence will decline. Burns are indeed dramatic, but they are often the last act of violence, not the first. Men who are likely to burn their wives are fixed in a pattern of violence that climaxes with the kerosene and a spark.

Furthermore, in light of these data, I think it is worthwhile to consider the idea that burns are not solely a function of dowry practices. If it were true that dowry causes bride burning, then dowry also produces emotional abuse, controlling behavior, slapping, and punching. And that argument simply does not follow: dowry cannot account for all violence against women. Dowry alone is not the cause of all the violence against women.

## Suicide By Self-Immolation

Data from the World Health Organization in 2009 shows that India's overall suicide rate is comparable to many other countries. A number of nations have suicide rates that are indeed very high internationally, and many of these countries are in Eastern Europe (Belarus 36.8 per 1,00,000; Lithuania 31.9; Russia 31.7). Sri Lanka's suicide rate was also relatively high at 31.7 per lakh population. Japan, Hungary, South Korea, and other Eastern European countries also had suicide rates over 20 per lakh population. India's rate was much lower at 10.7 per lakh, which was comparable to the United States (11.1), Ireland (10.6), Australia (10.5), Chile (10.4), and Singapore (10.3). Countries with very low suicide rates are Peru (0.9), Maldives (0.35), Iran (0.2), and Egypt (0.05). According to the Ministry of Home Affairs, India's rate has increased since these data were reported and in 2012 it was reported at 11.2 per 1 lakh. In that year, India witnessed 1,35,445 suicides (Ministry of Home Affairs 2013).

In all countries except China, men were more likely to commit suicide than women (World Health Organization 2009), and India followed the international pattern: men committed 65.3 per cent of all suicides. In most countries, however, men successfully completed suicide at rates three to seven times more than women. In India, the ratio between men and women was less than two to one, indicating that although the overall suicide rate in the country is not particularly high, the proportion of women killing themselves is among the highest in the world. Indian women's suicide rate is about 2.5 times higher than that of women in high-income countries, and suicide is projected to become the leading cause of death among women in the next few years (Patel et al. 2012).

As tragic as the figures on domestic violence are, the story worsens when we realize that a significant portion of female suicide is a product of distress and violence in their homes (Ellsberg et al. 2008; Garcia-Moreno 2009). When delving further into the ministry's data, we see that the suicide rate could conceivably be lower for women if domestic violence was not so severe in the subcontinent. According to the Ministry of Home Affairs (2013), in 2012, the causes of suicide differ between men and women in India. The two major causes of suicide for both men and women were listed as 'family problems', a nebulous category that does not specify identifiable reasons, and prolonged illness. Other problems listed as significant causes for suicide differ between the two sexes. In contrast to men whose causes of suicide are often economic – unemployment, poverty, and bankruptcy – women's suicides were disproportionately associated with other family matters such as divorce, dowry disputes, impotency (although who was infertile, the husband or the wife, was not necessarily known, the women bore the responsibility), and physical abuse. Many reports link domestic violence with women's suicide in what Dutta calls 'patriarchally propelled self-victimization' (2003: 26). Sometimes the violence committed by husbands is so brutal or the sex role expectations of women are so punitive that many women see no other way to escape except by killing themselves.

Men and women also differ in how they kill themselves. Hanging and poisoning, usually with pesticides, are the two most common methods for both sexes. Then there is a significant difference. As grotesque as it sounds, a common method that women use to take their own lives is by pouring kerosene on themselves and setting themselves on fire. Self-immolation is the third leading method of suicidal death among women in India and was the only method in which women outnumbered men: 64 per cent of self-immolations were women. In all other methods, such as guns and drowning, men outnumbered women, which is not surprising since men were almost twice as likely as women to take their own lives.

Self-immolation is a predominately female method of suicide – females commit about two of three burning suicides, and all age groups are vulnerable. In data reported by the ministry, there were 7,748 female burning suicides in 2012, and of those, 176 were girls 14 years or younger and 478 were women 60 years and older. Women aged 15–44 are particularly at risk; 6,168 women took their own lives by setting themselves on fire, and that's just in 2012. As with accidents, reported suicides may be murder disguised as suicide.

While men may not light these fires of self-destruction, they may share in a great deal of the responsibility. Suicide is not often an act of existential dilemma in which a person questions the meaning of life and his or her role in the universe. Instead, suicide is frequently an escape, a way out of a painful existence that perceives no end and no salvation. As gruesome as it sounds, these women would rather burn themselves alive than continue with the torture, humiliation, and suffering that they endure every day in the present and in the foreseeable future.

Not all women who set themselves afire are successful in taking their own lives. Many survive with scarred skin and disfigured appearances that are constant, visible reminders of their attempt to die and the miserable conditions that led to the act. They are often blamed for their own victimization and are treated with great prejudice by both family members and the general community. Suicide is primarily a social act, and for those who survive burns, the scars are socially interpreted and discredit the women who have survived both the tragedy of their lives and the horrendous pain of being burned. Is it true that women are to blame for attempting to take their lives when the pain of life is intolerable?

## Medical Remedies of Severe Disfigurement

In addition to the social and psychological aspects of kerosene and acid burns, burns such as those that cause severe disfigurement are serious medical conditions that require highly skilled emergency and follow-up care. Serious burns require emergency surgery, preferably in a specialized burn unit, in addition to multiple subsequent surgeries to repair damaged skin and restore appearance and functionality. Modern medical treatments, unfortunately, cannot fully restore pre-burn appearance. Scar tissue is inevitable, and depending on the severity and location of the burns, body parts can be damaged beyond repair. For the worst cases, 50 to 60 surgeries (even more in the most severe cases) can be required to return a victim to the best level of health and the most 'human' or natural appearance as possible.

Medical technology has produced three remedies for severe burns to the face: reconstruction, prostheses, and face transplantation. The latter two of these are not common in India or elsewhere in the world.

Before any of these remedies can be prescribed, however, victims of severe burns must undergo acute surgical care. Severe burns such as those caused by ignited kerosene and acid are traumatic medical events and must be treated as such. Emergency physicians and nurses, preferably in a specialized burn center, perform trauma care. Plastic surgeons are usually only contacted in consultation in this phase of treatment because comprehensive care is necessary to assess the risk of conditions beneath the skin. Physicians must determine if airways are clear and that breathing is unhindered, and they must check for intra-abdominal injuries, bleeding, and bone damage. As Renz and Cancio (2012: 615) state: 'The skin is intimately linked at a physiologic level to the function of every other organ system'. The more severe the burn, the more injurious the impact is likely to be on those systems. Immediate care is necessary because without it, patients have a far lower chance of recovery. Infections, pain, hypothermia, and organ failure are possible, if not probable. Acute surgeries are not designed to 'cure' burn patients, but to save their lives. These treatments are the platforms on which further treatments are built.

### Reconstruction

Once patients have stabilized following acute surgery, decisions are made as to the next step. Face reconstruction is the remedy choice in the vast majority of surgical responses to severe burns in both India and abroad. In these cases, the goal is to repair and rebuild the face with patients' own tissues in order to ameliorate cosmetic appearance and improve or restore functionality.

Patients may require as many as three scores or more reconstructive surgeries, which are usually conducted by plastic surgeons, in order to restore the highest level of attainable functionality and cosmetic appearance. Such a large number of surgeries is taxing on patients' well-being and are time-consuming, discomforting, and extremely costly. In order to achieve the best possible recovery, patients need continuous care and support from friends and family members to perform basic self-care tasks as well as financial maintenance as reconstruction patients are unable to work or tend to their families and themselves for extended periods of time because of pain and immobility.

Reconstructive techniques have other limitations as well. First, they typically leave patients with a patchwork appearance. It is never possible to match skin tone, even with skin from one's own body; therefore, when skin grafts heal, they will not match nearby skin tissues. Second, in many cases, surgeons cannot remove all the scar tissue, leaving some quite visible. Third, scars of stitching the grafts together often remain, adding slight borders to the quilt-like appearance of the mismatched coloration. Reconstructive surgeries, regardless of the skill of the surgeon, are almost always noticeable when performed on the face.

### *Prosthetics*

A second remedy option is facial prosthetics, false faces designed to replicate normal facial features and mask disfigurement. Prosthetics can be full-face masks or partial replicas, such as an eye and its surrounding tissues, engineered to blend with the rest of the natural face.

Facial prosthetics has an interesting modern history that merges theatrical art, plastic surgery, and the violence of warfare. Different from wars prior to 1914, World War I had particularly horrific and brutal physical consequences for the men who fought its battles. WWI was fought largely from trenches, which means that soldiers' faces and heads were unusually exposed to opposing gunfire. Wounds to the face were unprecedented in both frequency and severity, leaving thousands of young men horrifically disfigured. In addition, at that time in history, the weapons employed in WWI were the most powerful ever known and were capable of doing severe damage from a greater distance.

Once the war ended and these disfigured men returned to their homes, they found that medicine had no recourse for their condition. Soon, however, the idea arose to mask the wounds with static, nonmoving prosthetics, and artists collaborated with medical professionals to create various devices to help former soldiers look as normal as possible, or in many cases, to simply conceal the wounds. Known by war veterans as the Tin Nose Shop, The London General Hospital's Masks for Facial Disfigurement Department sought to provide the best possible plastic surgery and prosthetic care to disfigured war survivors. A similar facility operated in Paris's Latin Quarter and was known as the Studio for Portrait Masks in Paris and was administered by the Red Cross (Alexander 2007).

From this beginning, modern prosthetics remains an art and medical collaboration. The capability of prosthetics artists today can work wonders that were scarcely imaginable in the post-war years of the 1920s. Materials, paints, and anatomical knowledge are far superior to the past, and the prosthetics that artists create today are hardly noticeable in many cases, even at a close distance.

Despite the gains in techniques, prosthetics is not a perfect solution to disfigurement. Prosthetics artists are not widely available either geographically (there are not many of them) or financially (the cost can be quite high); therefore, prosthetics, if appropriate for a disfigured individual, may not be feasible. Second, prosthetics is not without limitations. Regardless of how real they may appear, the person wearing prosthetics looks somewhat unnatural in the region of the face covered by the prosthetics. The prosthesis cannot move, locking in a permanent expression. Therefore, the person may appear expressionless in the masked area. Although superior to disfigurement, prostheses are not often practical long-term remedies to severe burns. When prosthesis is possible, however, the results can be outstanding and provide a great benefit to the individual's self-esteem and sense of well-being.

## *Face Transplantation*

Face transplantation is a new, still experimental remedy for severe disfigurement. As of April 2016, 33 transplants have been conducted since 2005 when the first experiment was conducted in France. Transplantation is a complex surgery that requires a large operation theater and a sizeable team of physicians, nurses, and technicians. A face transplant requires a brain-dead donor whose family has agreed to allow surgeons to remove their deceased loved one's face and then transplant it onto the recipient whose disfigured face must be surgically extracted. The surgery is complicated and expensive and requires lifelong immunosuppression medications to prevent the recipient's body from rejecting the foreign tissue, which it sees as a biological 'invasion'. During the surgery, patients must undergo 15–20 hours of anesthesia, which carries its own risks and potential complications.

Immunosuppression comes with its own risks as well. First is the cost, which sums to tens of thousands of US dollars per year for life. Second, suppressing the immune system exposes the individual to heightened risks of infections and other illnesses.

Nevertheless, face transplantation has the potential to remedy severe disfigurement. Of the three medical options, transplantation is the best selection for restoring a normal, unadulterated appearance, and it could relieve many if not most of the functional impairments that a disfigured person my experience due to the fire, trauma, or disease that caused the face to become disfigured. Recipients' appearance is a blend of their pre-disfigured face and that of the donor, depending on how much donor tissue is transplanted. Although transplantation is the best choice to recreate a normal appearance, the procedure is not yet sufficiently advanced for widespread use. Techniques are still improving, and, as has been learned in the early years of the surgery, patients must be carefully screened for suitability. In other words, not everyone who is severely disfigured is an appropriate candidate. Some may not have sufficient bone, muscular, and neurological health to receive and connect to the new facial tissues, while others may not have the psychological recourses necessary to comply to medical orders following surgery or to handle the reality of having another person's face. Perhaps the primary problem with face transplantation, however, is the immunosuppression drugs required to prevent tissue rejection. These medicines are very strong and expensive and require strict compliance protocols.

To date, face transplantation is not available in India. Although that is likely to change in the future because of advances in plastic and microsurgery in India, the costs of both surgery and lifelong immunosuppression are prohibitive to the vast majority of Indians. Face transplantation, at least at this time, is not a viable option in the country.

In summary, all of the medical treatments of severe facial burns are expensive and complex, and they still do not restore the victim of burns to a completely 'normal' appearance. The quality of prostheses has improved immensely, but prostheses require expensive artistic and medical skills and, though they have become more aesthetically pleasing, they do not allow any facial expression or function. Furthermore, the disfigurement remains; it is simply hidden behind the false face. Any pain associated with the scars remains as well. Transplantations may restore some sense of normalcy in that the burned tissue can be replaced and the suture scars hidden by hair and clothing. However, transplantation is an extremely expensive surgery that is still in experimental stages. Plus, lifelong needs for costly antirejection medications, which present their own medical problems, make face transplantation impractical and prohibitive for most, if not all, severely disfigured women in India.

Surgical reconstruction, therefore, continues to be the most likely medical response to severe burns. Reconstruction, common as it is in the case of burns, is not a simple procedure. In fact, it is not one procedure. As already mentioned, most severe burn victims require several if not scores of surgeries because severe burn conditions typically require surgeons to work on different parts of the face in separate surgeries. In most cases, it cannot all be done at once. Usually surgeons will conduct emergency plastic surgery and microsurgery immediately after the burn to remove dead tissue and graft live tissue from other parts of the body, which also leaves painful wounds at the site of the donation. These operations focus on saving lives and minimal functional and aesthetic restoration. In the West, these surgeries are usually followed by further improvements to functionality and cosmetic surgeries that enhance appearance. In India, many, if not most, burn victims do not receive treatment beyond the immediate, life-saving interventions. Furthermore, patients of reconstruction often appear to have patchwork appearance in addition to scars and misshaped features.

The purpose of this brief description of medical responses to facial burns is to show that the outcomes of severe burns are permanent. The best medicine and surgical techniques cannot restore an individual's pre-burn appearance. Ears and noses cannot be reconstructed in a way that looks 'right', and eyelids cannot be rebuilt at all. Men and women who are burned to this degree cannot hide their features from the view of other people. The wounds are obvious, and they cause survivors to stand out as different, subjecting them to the process of 'othering' in which they are under the threat of becoming judged and evaluated against normative expectations of appearance. The scars are signs to both strangers and people with whom they have relationships that something is not right, and as shall be seen in the next chapter, the permanence of burn scars has a highly negative impact on victims' social lives.

## Conclusion

This chapter veers from the theoretical aspects of violence against women to show various aspects of burns such as the historical considerations of burning women, incidence and prevalence, the injuries and treatments from burns, and the social patterns and context in which burns occur. The chapter concluded by noting the permanence of burn wounds, and although that sounds like stating the obvious, it is important to remember because the wounds are inflicted upon these women by their husbands and not the result of an accident. Given what will happen to women once they become 'burned women', it is all the more important to remember that this life circumstance is not of their choosing, it is victimization that will last the duration of their lives.

As shown in Chapter 2, the status of women in the subcontinent is quite poor. Study after study on gender in India reports great differentials in well-being and quality of life between men and women. These differences are found in virtually all aspects of life: health, education, literacy, economic participation, and political engagement. In addition, women suffer high rates of domestic violence and politically motivated violence.[3]

Research is clear that burn violence is not a single or isolated attack on victims. There is almost always a context of other violence or marital conflict that precedes the attack. It seems convenient to blame dowry for 'bride burning'; however, I contend that targeting dowry is an overly simplistic explanation, especially in light of research that indicates that dowry problems are frequently not present in marriages where burns occur (Kumar et al. 2014). Dowry may explain some cases, but it may be a mistake to blame all such violence on this cultural practice.

Burn attacks as well as other forms of violence against women are not regularly adjudicated in Indian courts, which serves to reinforce inequalities in social power. Peck (2012) found that in 2008 Indian courts convicted 1,948 men of dowry deaths, many of which were committed by burning. These same courts, however, acquitted 3,876 men accused of murdering their wives. Violence and the threat of violence hold women in check and deny them access to self-expression, actualization, and individual liberty.

More to the point, burn violence suggests equating femaleness with nothingness.

Women who are not wanted are often subjected to cleansing through fire or acid in a symbolic ritual with two possible desired results: a restoration of purity or eradication from the earth. Burning can accomplish both. Turning women to ashes is more than an assault; it is a symbolic, if not real, attempt to cremate them while they are still alive – to destroy the vessel of life, yet holding the soul in contempt. But this is a very different symbolic ritual from cremation and sati, which is also about purity. Bride burning shows disdain and disregard for the living female body.

For those women who survive, as will be seen in the next chapter, life is routinely made difficult because of the assault. Because of their wounds, they are stigmatized and often held in disdain. They are not fully burned; the burn is incomplete, which is indicated by their survival. Therefore, they are marked as tainted not solely because their bodies do not fit the feminine ideal, but also, as we shall see, there exists an added level of disdain that ventures deeper than their blemished skin: sense of contempt and disgust pervades their relationships with other people.

## Notes

1. The 5 million estimate is derived through a simple arithmetic. From various demographic sources, I estimated the number of women aged 18 and older to be about 35,00,00,000 in 2006. I multiplied that figure by 0.019, the rate of burned survivors discovered by the random sample. The actual product is about 7.5 million, but allowing women not yet married (students, for example), those not otherwise in the marriage pool (incarcerated and chronically ill or disabled), and so forth renders 50,00,000. This figure is little more than an 'educated guess' and was not meant to be the precise prevalence of deliberate burns.

2. Less severe violence is defined as violence that is less likely to cause injury. The descriptive 'less severe' does not suggest minimizing the violence, but represents a qualitative difference in violence that can cause physical harm. Examples of more severe violence include the use of weapons and, of course, burning.
3. For the present purposes, examples of politically motivated violence include honor killings and attacks on women to discredit them communally, such as in the Gujarat riots.

# 4

# Stigma[1]

> Eighteen goddess-like daughters are not equal to one son with a hump.
>
> —Indian saying

When a woman is burned, the attack is only the beginning of a long and painful journey through life. Following the physical pain of the burns, the surgeries, and the subsequent scarring, comes the worst part: living with disfigurement. Like their disfigured counterparts in the West, severely disfigured women in India are set aside from regular society and thrown into a smaller social world where they are often depressed, anxious, and alone. In India, however, severely scarred women suffer a crueler fate in which basic survival is a challenge, and the quest for respect is rarely fulfilled. People living with disabilities are routinely singled out as unfit or undesirable; however, few, if any, physical differences are as subject to such severe social rejection as disfigurement. There is something unique about the face that makes its loss so very devastating.

As discussed in Chapter 1, the face is a complex and subjective part of the human body that serves as a main point of intersection between an individual and social sentiment in relationships with other people. Central to individual identification and sexual attraction, the face is essentially a sign declaring the social markers of our status in society. In addition, the face can communicate emotions such as fear and anger, shame and embarrassment, and happiness and joy, and contains the cluster of senses of sight, smell, taste, hearing, and touch. While we use our faces to send symbolic messages, we also deduce from others' expressions their moods and motivations. 'Reading' facial expressions provides critical information for understanding a social situation and imputing individual and social desires. Echoing Chapter 1, the face can be considered the focal point of human life, a reality that becomes clear when we assess how 'society' treats people whose faces are disfigured by trauma or disease.

Appearance dominates peoples' interpretations of disfigured persons, whose unusual looks become their defining feature and carry a sharply negative connotation. Studies on disfigurement in North America and Europe demonstrate that disfigurement is linked to prejudice, discrimination, stereotyping, and social isolation. Individuals who are disfigured are often treated disrespectfully and are relatively socially powerless when compared to 'normal looking' individuals (Pruzinsky 1992).

Disfigured people are subject to stigma, a process of discrediting a person or group by virtue of possessing some distinguishing characteristic. Stigma is expressed in a number of ways: economic discrimination, being ostracized from most normative social relationships and opportunities, routine disrespect, and social powerlessness (Pruzinsky 1992; Robinson 1997). Here are a few examples: Studies have found that job recruiters negatively perceive facially disfigured applicants and hold an adverse bias of their work-related skills (Stevenage and McKay 1999); pedestrians stand further away from a disfigured person while waiting to cross a street (Rumsey, Bull, and Gahagan 1982); people spend less time with and give less money to disfigured charity workers (Bull and Stevens 1981); users of public transportation sit farther from disfigured than non-disfigured riders (Houston and Bull 1994); and teachers' academic expectations of disfigured children are lower than for non-disfigured pupils (Walters 1997). Life after being burned carries a stigma that many victims say is the real pain of the whole affair.

## Stigma

Stigma is a cornerstone concept in sociology and is defined as a physical or social attribute that devalues a person's social identity and disqualifies him or her from complete social acceptance (Goffman 1963). This attribute, especially if visible, is one that is interpreted in such a way that disgraces the individual. Because the characteristic or 'mark' carries high social valence, it becomes an individual's 'master status', the attribute that takes priority over all others in the formation of a person's social identity and has the most influence during interactions with others.

Stigma theory also places into perspective the clinical and survey research that consistently reports an association between facial deformity and psychological stress and a less than desirable quality of life (Pruzinsky 1992; Rumsey et al. 2004). Facially disfigured individuals are frequently shut-ins, hiding from social relationships that others take for granted. They face a number of psychological problems, such as social anxiety, lowered self-confidence and self-esteem, negative self-image, depression, alcohol abuse, and marital problems (Levine et al. 2005; Pruzinsky et al. 2005; Robinson 1997; Rumsey et al. 2004). These conditions are often mutually reinforcing and lead an individual into further seclusion and anxiety when relating to other people. The more frequently that disfigured people encounter startled responses, avoiding glances, and other off-putting messages in the social world, the more likely they are to avoid social interactions altogether.

More often than not, they will develop a sense of self that reflects this social rejection.

In sociology, minority group status is assigned to groups that possess a primary and defining characteristic (e.g. race, sexual orientation, or physical state) that distinguishes them from a more powerful group that does not have the characteristic. This distinguishing mark is stereotyped and stigmatized and identifies an individual as a member of a group whose 'place' in society is subordinate and whose social entitlements are restricted. Usually we think of minority status in terms of racial and ethnic groups, but sociologists consider all disenfranchised groups, including people with physical disabilities or differences, minorities as well.

In this way of thinking, disfigurement qualifies as a minority-defining characteristic. In the case of disfigurement due to burns, however, a person is not born into the minority or marginalized status. Instead, the status is ascribed after the burn assault. Why this change in appearance seemingly automatically carries stigma in virtually all cultures is not well understood and poses a number of questions: How does disfigurement change the social conventions of human relationships? Why are the rules of interaction modified when a person becomes disfigured? Why are people often startled when they see a disfigured person?

To begin to answer these questions, more on stigma theory is in order. The word 'stigma' finds its origins in ancient Greek. Derived from the root *stizein*, meaning to mark or tattoo, the Greek word *stigma* (plural *stigmata*) represented a mark made with a sharp stick or tattooing tool to puncture or brand slaves to show they were in the service of the temple or master to which they were bonded. A marking also was applied to morally corrupt persons such as criminals or runaway slaves (Falk 2001). The first known English usage of 'stigma' is found in the late 16th century where the term referred to a mark of disgrace made on the skin made by a hot iron. Ironically, during the medieval period the term also took on Christian religious significance and referred to physical manifestations of the suffering of Jesus Christ. Having such signs, or stigmata, appear on the body indicated holy grace.

Since the 1500s, the word has maintained its original Greek meaning; however, the scope of the concept has evolved to include more statuses than slavery and more infractions than major criminal violations than that found among the early Greeks. Furthermore, stigmas are no longer physically imposed on targets but constitute the very attributes themselves. Race and ethnicity, sex and sexuality, various qualities of ill health especially mental health, and physical ability and appearance, including facial disfigurement, also came to be the subject of stigmatization. Those status and physical qualities have become defined as the stigma. No forced additional cut, brand, or tattoo was necessary.

Consequently when social scientists talk about stigma, they are referring to a multidimensional concept, and many theoretical and conceptual schemes have been proffered to account for the variance in the types of the attributes that are subject to discrediting and the social process by which the stigmatization occurs. The ideas of two theorists, Gerhard Falk and Erving Goffman, are particularly relevant to furthering our understanding of disfigurement stigma.

Falk situates stigma in a Durkheimian functionalist context where a stigma serves to heighten a sense of community and solidarity. By targeting and labeling outsiders who violate key mores as morally corrupt or tainted, the insiders are compelled to bond and form the group's definition of what is right, moral, and desirable. Falk argued that stigma lies in the discrepancy between core values and perceived deviation of those values (Falk 2001).

For Falk, stigma has two forms: existential stigma and achieved stigma. Existential or societal stigma is one in which the target, the stigmatized person, did not cause or had little control over. It is an attribute that violates consensus and takes the form of qualities inherent in the target's essential being. Examples of Falk's existential stigma are age, sex, sexual orientation, and race and ethnicity. Achieved stigma, which he also called situational, refers to a stigma attached to an actual deed acted out by the target; it is related to the conduct of the target person and groups. Alcoholism and criminal behavior serve as examples. When core expectations of behavior and social desirability are violated, the group senses the deviants to be threatening to its ability to function cohesively and reacts by discrediting them. Thus, rule-breaking behavior and conformity are maintained within acceptable limits and the social group continues to engage in a harmonious and systematic fashion.

Falk's approach helps understand disfigurement stigma in that it illustrates the emotional boundaries of values within groups. In other words, values have emotional subtexts, and emotions are triggered when core values are violated, causing people to rally together to resist the violators. These values, of course, change as the discourse of society changes throughout the tides of history. Each period of history, as defined by time and space, has its own views of the essential qualities of human character, and each social location has those people who feel they have identified the true essence or cause of whatever the stigmatized mark may be. One can, for instance, 'know' the true cause of mental illness or that a particular ethnic group is biologically inferior or that women lack the mental capabilities of men. These so-called truths change and vary by social grouping, which reminds us that essentialist thinking is actually socially constructed and reminds us that that which constitutes reality is neither finite nor permanent.

Falk's approach does not address a number of important questions about stigma. For example, the Durkheimian framework does not answer many questions about the nature of the power that originates and enforces the stigma. What is the origin of those norms and values that are perceived to be violated, and who has the social legitimacy to stigmatize others? At another level of analysis, how does being stigmatized affect one's sense of self? How do people manage stigma within the context of the norms and values that they have broken, or perceived to have broken, by others? What are symbolic meanings of the rules that are broken? That is, rules are violated routinely; therefore, why does deviant behavior or status result in stigma in some situations and among some people and groups while not in others?

The sociologist Erving Goffman's approach to stigmatization helps us resolve those questions. For Goffman, stigma occurs in the conduct of everyday behavior and exists in the context of symbolic meanings held by a social group. Stigma has symbolic meaning that is derived from expectations of what life, and people, should be like. Goffman contended that stigma is first grounded in the gap between 'virtual social identity' and 'actual social identity'. Virtual identity is the general socially shared idea of what a person should be. Actual identity, on the other hand, is what a person actually is. When there is a discrepancy between the two identities, that is, when there is a difference between how society characterizes a social ideal and the attributes the person actually possesses, stigma occurs, and at that point, interaction between stigmatizers and the stigmatized changes.

Stigma, therefore, is a discrediting mark that is assigned to individuals and groups and distinguishes them from those who conform to the ideal or virtual social identity; stigmatization, consequently, is the social process in which a person (or group) migrates from 'a whole and usual person to a tainted discounted one' (Goffman 1963: 3). The qualities that stray from the ideal are negatively labeled to ensure the persons with those qualities are marginalized, and once defined as alien, stigmatized persons can be kept at a safe distance from the core culture.

Goffman argued that individuals who are targets of stigma are first perceived as people who would have been received 'normally' in ordinary social interactions, meaning that stigmatizers would have treated the person with the attribute as if there were no distinguishing characteristic. However, stigmatized individuals possess a trait or attribute that turns the attention of others to a peculiar or differentiating attribute. For Goffman, there are three such classes of attributes. The first is admonitions of the body, which takes the form of deformities, levels of attractiveness, and body shape. Blemishes on character are the second category of stigmatized attributes. Here Goffman is describing stigma levied at people with domineering or unnatural passions or rigid or treacherous beliefs. He includes in this category suicidal behavior, criminal behavior, addictions, and homosexuality. Goffman's third category is known as tribal stigma, which targets people of particular ethnic and racial groups simply by virtue of being born into those groups. He said that this stigma is transmitted through lineage and 'equally contaminates all members of a family' (1963: 14).

Stigma is also rooted in the source of the attribute that discredits an individual or group. In this regard, Goffman made the distinction between two kinds of stigmas: discredited and discreditable. Discreditable stigma refers to those who believe their stigma is not known or perceivable by others. Stigmas based on conduct, for instance, are discreditable until a behavior is revealed. Being in a stigmatized religion or marital status, such as being divorced, for example, that does not necessarily have visible identifiers are discreditable; that is, the bearer can conceal the stigmatized characteristic and interact without others acting on the knowledge of the stigmatized mark. Character blemishes, such as being a former convict or having a mental illness, are often discreditable statuses. Unless the person's status is revealed publicly, he or she can often 'pass', which means to maintain a 'normal' social identity, one without the taint. Once a discreditable attribute is known and hence discredited, social interaction and social definitions of the person will change to accommodate the stigma.

Discredited stigma refers to those individuals and groups who presume their identity is known and obvious to others. A discredited identity, such as physical and tribal stigmas, is based on a visual attribute that is not easily concealed. For example, being confined to a wheel chair and being a member of racial group in which membership is based on a readily identifiable external feature such as skin color can often become discredited. These attributes are easy for others to see and to expose for judgment. Discredited stigmas force people to respond to the gap between what is and what ought to be via what Goffman called covering. Covering is behavior that seeks to reduce tension during social interactions. Because the stigma is visible or the person's identity is made public, the stigmatized person cannot pass as a 'normal' and thus attempts to make the stigma as unobtrusive as possible. They will hide the mark and/or alter their behavior to minimize the emotional charge that the attribute introduces into the social exchange. Severely disfigured women, for example, will use cosmetics and veils or other clothing to cover their facial features. They often avoid eye contact and face-to-face interaction with other people.

### Stigma and Social Conflict

Sociologists have long believed that social identity is facilitated by the presence of outsiders, social groups that differ from one's own culture or break social rules. Seemingly paradoxical, focusing on how 'others' are different from us reinforces cohesiveness within and loyalty to our own group. That is, outsiders and rule breakers strengthen conformity to social ideals and values. Our sense of community is promoted when we can judge others unfit and outside the boundaries of our own group. In other words, creating a 'them' (who are 'wrong') defines the 'we' (who are 'right').

Despite sounding nice and integrative, in-group bonding (and therefore out-group exclusion) often creates social tension and open conflict. Rather than promoting idyllic social cohesion, strictly drawn social boundaries are typically anxious and because they are based on rules of exclusion, construct groups of people who are denied some of the social benefits of the in-group. When differences between groups are particularly stressful, we usually collapse or retreat to the comforts of the familiarity of our own group; we feel safe from the threats, real or perceived, that 'different' people present.

For people and groups to do this requires the out-group to have an identifying characteristic, preferably one that is visible and easily distinguishes the others as being outside the parameters of the home group identity. Excluding others, however, requires an ideology or belief that defines others' differences as objectionable and then justifies and rationalizes the undesirability of those differences. This belief system 'explains' why the distinguishing characteristic is bad and unworthy and does so within the political and cultural context of the times. Classic examples include racist pseudo-science used in the past to justify racial segregation in the United States, religious beliefs that contributed to the basis of rationalizing the caste structure in India, and sexist arguments that contend inherent differences between men and women justify female subordinance. To support these beliefs, the differences, which for all practical purposes are superficial, are accentuated, given far more importance than they merit, and are stereotyped and stigmatized as highly unattractive and distasteful.

Outsiders are assigned to a cultural category that damages their material, social, and psychological well-being (Kroska and Harkness 2006). Members of a society's minority groups, which includes individuals with mental illness, disabilities, and severe disfigurement, generally suffer higher unemployment, receive less education, and experience feelings of alienation, demoralization, and minimalization (Link 1987). Outsiders are rated as categorically different, and frequently rated as tainted or of lesser value by the guiding ideology. In other words, stigma is a socially constructed process, occurring within a broad social and political milieu.

Any given stigma may be guided and informed by social norms and values, but it is expressed in the context of daily social encounters. Whereas psychological approaches emphasize individual characteristics and psychological adjustment to stigma and stigma as a static feature (Link and Phelan 2001), sociological theories conceptualize stigma as a dynamic process of labeling and ascription that occurs within the broader system of values, power, and social control (Parker and Aggleton 2003) in which social groups invent and perpetuate rules of social exclusion and marginalization. As Parker and Aggleton aptly state, stigma 'always has a history which influences when it appears and the form it takes' (2003: 17).

*Stigma and Moral Authority:* Central to this 'history' is the role of moral experience in defining a characteristic as shameful and how that mark becomes embedded in the moral life of sufferers (Yang et al. 2007). Stigma occurs in a stigmatized person's immediate social milieu within which daily life and moral experiences are played out. For Yang et al. (2007), these local worlds are social arenas with high stakes, where status, money, relationships, life chances, work, and health are won and lost. The local world is the social place for what matters most in ordinary people's lives, thus defining individuals' and groups' moral experience.

Yang et al.'s theory, which stems from a long-neglected hypothesis of Goffman's, contends that stigma is a moral issue because the stigmatized condition threatens what really matters in life. Focusing on 'lived or social experience' (2007: 1528) identifies not only that of the upmost importance in life, but also that which most threatens life's essentials. Stigma is a pragmatic response to menace and the unknown, and constitutes the 'existential and moral experience that one is being threatened' (Yang et al. 2007: 1528). Stigma is thus a sub-set within the larger class of social discrimination where the social exclusion attached to the stigmatized mark functions as an indicator of a threat to some moral imperative that regulates the affairs of everyday life. It is a discrimination based less on exploitation, but on fear of disrupting the most fundamental sense of 'normality'.

## Stigma Theory and Disfigurement

If a characteristic of a person or group is stigmatized because it is threatening to the moral sentiments of a group, then what does disfigurement threaten? And if the idea driving stigma is to keep the 'bad' separated from the 'good', what is inherently 'bad' about a disfigured facial appearance?

Below I will describe a study carried out in a large city in South India that sought to answer these questions. By examining the experiences of a number of women whose lives are largely defined by their appearance, I sought to extract themes that point toward the origins of stigma. As shall be shown, women who are disfigured are indeed stigmatized by others, and the consequences of this stigma are not insignificant. From the descriptions of their experiences, I will attempt to draw theoretical conclusions about the nature of disfigurement stigma in India.

### How the Study Was Conducted

Data for this study were collected from a judgmental sample organized by a nongovernmental social service agency that provides a wide array of services to disadvantaged women in a large city in southern India. Judgmental sampling is a nonrandom strategy that allows researchers to use their judgment in selecting cases that are considered typical of the population under study. Cases are selected based on the decision that they are exemplar representatives of the inclusion criteria. Given that victims of fire assaults are neither recorded nor easily accessible and are geographically dispersed, a judgmental, or purposeful, sampling technique was used to identify women who met the following inclusion criteria: the women must be disfigured due to an attack by their husbands; disfigurement must be easily visible; and the disfigurement must be at least partially facial. (The women had varying degrees of disfigurement, but no attempt was made to measure the amount of scarred body tissue each woman possessed.) Unsuccessful suicide by self-immolation, as mentioned earlier, is not uncommon in India and leaves scars and disfigurations that differ little than those resulting from attacks. Given that suicide itself carries stigma that might confound others' interpretation of disfigurement due to domestic violence, women disfigured by an attempt to take their own lives were excluded from the study group.

Because disfigured women, whose appearance is the result of violence, are more often than not still living with or near the person who attempted to murder them, and are severely discriminated against, they are difficult to identify. In addition, most cannot often admit publicly that their husbands attacked them, and few have the luxury to move about freely. Therefore, I relied upon the judgment of a social worker employed at the agency to select women who fit my purpose for conducting the study – that is, they were qualified, were reasonably safe from the backlash of others who might react to their participation with anger, and best fit the purpose of the study.

The social worker who assisted in data collection provides domestic violence awareness education to communities and basic social support services to women victims of violence. Following our discussions of the sampling protocol, she contacted women whom she knew directly or indirectly from her assigned caseload and invited them to participate in the study. During this phase of sampling, while I met four potential participants to acclimatize myself to the conditions of the study, all the women were interviewed by the social worker before they were asked to participate in the study. From these interviews, several women were rejected for the following reasons: disfigurement was due to a suicide attempt; scars were not facial; emotional fragility; or safety concerns.

In light of the sensitivity of the women's experiences, no identifying or demographic data were collected. All but two of the women who agreed to participate continued to live with or near their assailants; thus, there were potential safety issues concerning participation for most of the women involved.

Remembering the emotional distress I experienced from my encounter with 'Gita', which was discussed in the Preface, I made the study as anonymous as possible and did not ask for any identifying information.[2] Seeing firsthand the fear Gita and her relatives had and the fresh wounds on her arms and torso, I could hardly imagine what would have happened to her if her husband knew that she spoke to me. The risks she took by merely leaving her house were extraordinary. Had something gone wrong and it became known that Gita was physically punished for the simple act of telling her story to me; I would have never forgiven myself.

Therefore, I vowed to take more cautions than usual to protect the identity of the study's volunteer participants. I simply referred to each participant by number in my notes and translations, and I gathered little demographic data.

Nonetheless, a few characteristics of the sample can be described. Most of the participants volunteered their ages at the beginning of the discussions, the youngest was 19 and the eldest was 51. The women were of lower caste origins, indicating they were from low to modest income families. None, however, came from extreme poverty, at least as it is defined in India, or was destitute. Their financial and material support was derived from various sources including their families of origin, in-laws, or employment, most of which was marginal. Those employed worked as servants or street-side vendors. Husbands provided little support for their disfigured wives and children. None of the women was legally divorced, and all had children and were at least two years removed from the disfiguring assault.

The sample of 21 women was divided into two focus groups (10 in one group and 11 in the second). The focus group technique was deemed the most appropriate tool of choice for data collection for this study due to its effectiveness in exploring sensitive topics; researchers have shown that peer discussion groups are efficacious in helping participants feel more comfortable and less judged in sharing their thoughts and experiences (Morgan 1996). Morgan further contends that focus groups are a particularly effective research strategy when working with illiterate persons or those with minimal language skills. More specific to the present study, Mehta (2011) contends that focus groups are particularly effective in Asia, where educational levels may be low and that the technique is a more suitable approach for gathering information than self-administered questionnaires. Sharing life stories among peers, furthermore, brings a sense of social and psychological comfort via validation, support, and simply being taken seriously.

Prior to convening the focus groups, I met with the assisting social workers to review the nature of the study, the expectations for the process of the data collection, and the meaning of the questions. Minor adjustments to the original interview questions were made to reduce awkward translations. The focus group discussions were loosely structured to allow the participants freedom to tell their stories and to interact with each other. Certain questions were asked of both groups, but for the most part, the leader and I used prompts and follow-up questions to maintain the flow of the conversation.

Each focus group discussion lasted about 90 minutes and was attended by the researcher, a Tamil-speaking colleague, and two social workers employed at the agency. The meetings were held in a comfortable room in the organization's offices. One of the social workers led the discussions in Tamil and the other recorded notes in Tamil and English. The social workers translated and transcribed the discussions with the aid of my colleague.

Both groups had lively discussions that elicited a wide-range of emotions and content. Although the participants did not know each other, most gave their life stories comfortably and later stated their appreciation for the opportunity to discuss what many called the greatest tragedy of their lives. For almost all of the participants, this was the first occasion to talk about the events and pain in their lives following the assaults that disfigured them. The groups provided an outlet for these victims of violence to relate and somewhat make public their personal biographies and sorrows.

The women were read a statement in Tamil, their native language, informing them of their rights as research subjects. All participants provided consent to participate and be recorded. Once the recordings were translated into English and transcribed, the tapes were destroyed. Participants' names and other identifying information were not recorded. Lunch was provided as compensation for their time and participation.

*Study Limitations:* This study contains limitations that restrict its robustness and utility. First, the study is limited by sample selection constraints. Disfigured people are a small and hard to reach population, making large and random samples, and therefore generalizations impossible. The sample of disfigured women studied here is select. The women were recruited by an organization that provided support to the women. Although the sample met the study's inclusion criteria of having been burned by fire in a domestic assault and having resulting scars that are visible and facial, the women were known to the agency whose social workers who recruited them, which may present selection bias. For example, there was little variance in class/caste and education status, factors that may affect the forms stigma take.

Second, projections of the intent of the people who stigmatize were based on evidence gained by victims of stigmatization. Therefore, there is the possibility that research on the stigmatizers would yield results different from those presented here.

Direct quotes are presented as translated. Although the English is 'rough', the original translation was kept as a way of capturing the intent of the speaker. The translator, a Tamil speaker, understood the sentiments that the women in groups were conveying. 'Translating the translation' into more proper English, I feared, might impose unintended ideas on each speaker. The assumption is that the Tamil-speaking translator was culturally in tune with the speakers' real meaning and expressed it better than I could.

## *What Disfigurement Stigma Looks Like*

Before addressing the theoretical questions regarding the moral underpinning of stigma, the study was required to establish the existence of disfigurement stigma. Following the determination of the stigma, the analysis then moved toward identifying themes of moral sentiments within the context of the general stigma.

*The Presence of Stigma:* The data extracted from the focus groups support literature on samples in the United States and Britain that has demonstrated that disfigured women confront stigmatic responses from others in their everyday lives (c.f. Robinson 1997). All the discussants reported continuous, negative, humiliating, and hostile reactions to their appearance, and having been excluded from family affairs, denied employment, and publicly avoided. The maltreatment began on a daily basis immediately upon returning home from the hospitals where they underwent emergency plastic and reconstructive surgery and other treatments for severe burns. As one woman summarized the lives of disfigured women, 'We suffer a lot'.

Similar to reports on disfigured persons in the United States and United Kingdom, disfigured Indian women must handle other people staring at them, reacting with surprise to their appearance, asking unwanted and intrusive questions about the cause of their disfigurement, and speaking harshly and abusively to them. People routinely maintain greater distance from disfigured women than non-disfigured persons in public places such as buses, busy streets, and in shops, according to participants in both focus groups. From the women's perspective, the large majority of people with whom they have social contact have an off-putting, even harsh, connotation of disfigurement. Another woman in one of the groups said that people often say to her, 'Why don't you just die?'

As Yang et al.'s (2007) stigma theory suggests, the stigma the women face occurs in everyday social interaction. The women in the focus groups stated that others tell them that they are not good people and have no dignity, often calling them prostitutes or some similarly derogatory epithet. In light of these attitudes, the women are impelled to alter their behavior, making conventional social rules difficult to follow.

Each woman in the groups asserted further that the majority of people they encounter avoid contact with them. The women know that their appearance makes others feel uncomfortable, and a few reported that they will excuse themselves from a social situation in order to spare the other person the embarrassment of being seen with a disfigured person. Ordinary and mundane conversations and situations with disfigured women can easily be quite tense. Onc woman described a visit to another's home:

> I went to a neighbor's house to watch television, but the lady in that house asked me to go away as her husband and children will come and they may fear seeing me.

A large portion of the women in the groups stated that they are perceived as unpredictable and even dangerous. Because they are generally feared, they are blamed for the mistakes and problems that occur in the family and neighborhood. This generalized fear disrupts routines and forces adjustments in everyday routine. For example, one woman described that her appearance interrupted her extended family's kitchen habits because other women in the household would not touch the tableware from which she ate and drank, which resulted in two separate sets of dish-washing activities at each meal, every day.

Disruptions to everyday life occur outside the home as well. The presence of disfigured women, as they testified, disrupts the flow of pedestrian traffic on sidewalks, as people routinely veer off their course to avoid them, thus upsetting the rhythm, and the moods, of other walkers. Similarly one woman, a flower vendor, made other shopkeepers feel uneasy and apprehensive if she set up her business nearby. Other shopkeepers routinely coerce her to relocate for fear that people would not shop at their own businesses because they would have to come in proximity to a disfigured vendor. The shopkeepers would say to potential customers, according to the woman in the focus group, 'Don't buy flowers from her. She is burnt'.

The women conveyed other disruptions to daily life that were more serious in nature. For example, one woman told of the difficulty she had giving birth in a local hospital. The attending physician did not want to be bothered to deliver her child. When she approached the end of her labor, she stated that the doctor, in a perturbed manner, said, 'Why do you need this business? Do you think you are beautiful?'

The women realize that disfigurement has changed their roles in the conduct of everyday life, although they do not necessarily understand the reasons. Some believe that others think of them as impure, though not necessarily in the religious sense, or contaminated with infectious leprosy. Mostly, however, the women agree that the source of their discrimination in daily life is the perception that disfigurement has reduced their ability to perform everyday tasks. Almost all reported having been called 'cheap' (*kevalamana*), which suggests that their value is low and that they can be easily replaced.

The women did not report examples of chastisement connected to their functional abilities; all negative reactions were related to their appearance and came from strangers, acquaintances, and family members. Clearly the women's facial appearance had become a mark of stigma and exposed them to difficult social relationships that had not existed before their attacks. Returning to the purpose of the present study, given that stigma against disfigurement exists in everyday interaction, how, as Yang et al.'s (2007) theory suggests, is disfigurement threatening? What does disfigurement challenge in the scope of everyday life in India?

Following the conclusion that disfigurement stigma exists, qualitative analysis of the texts of the focus groups sought to identify normative patterns of moral threat related to disfigurement, and two such themes were extracted. As Yang et al. (2007) suggest, these stigma patterns are attached to the norms and values that govern everyday behavior and sentiments in India. The two themes of stigma found in these data are (1) threats to the values and practices of family rules and expectations, and (2) threats to religious sensibilities.

*Threats to Family Life:* The first emerging theme within these data is that disfigured women are threatening to the family in general and mothering in particular. Women in the study lived in three household types: some had returned to their families of origin; others continued to live with their husbands' families; and a few lived on their own. Of the women living with families of origin or in in-laws' households, all but one resided in a segregated setting apart from the rest of the family. One woman, for instance, lived in a single-room thatch hut on the roof of a three-story multifamily dwelling. Her husband's family occupied the first floor. A number of women continued an interpersonal and even sexual relationship with their husbands, including two cases where the husband had taken another wife. These women stated that these relationships were largely unpleasant emotionally and occasionally physically and sexually abusive.

Every woman in the two groups stated that they had lost status, rights, and privileges within their extended families. Except for women living independently as heads of household, the study participants rarely were allowed to contribute to family decision-making and were habitually minimized and marginalized. One woman said that:

> if a quarrel happens (in the family), the women start talking about my disfigured skin. They use harsh words like, 'why are you arguing with us? You don't even have the status to talk with us. You are not full-fledged. You are burnt!'

Another said, 'I stay at home. People make fun of me calling me 'The Burnt' (*karugeya*)'. A third woman described what happens when she goes to her parents' home:

> My family members are very suspicious. Even if I come and stand outside my house they will ask me, 'Why are you standing here? Who are you waiting to see?'

The questions, as reported by the woman, were voiced in anger.

For another woman in the sample, her family's rejection was especially pernicious. Her own family facilitated arranging a second marriage for her husband (the person who allegedly set her on fire) and provided little to no support for her and her children. The woman's parents held the assumption that the husband was either not at fault or was justified in his actions because of their daughter's failures as a wife and mother. They consequently felt obliged to help him, but not her.

In fact, in every case of attack by fire reported by these women, the female victims were held accountable to varying degrees. Most were accused of having extramarital affairs, while others were deemed inefficient or ineffective as wives and mothers. The men were rarely held responsible for their actions, according to the women. One husband was in hiding from the police. Only one offending husband had been arrested, and although his wife was grossly disfigured (the most severely disfigured of the sample), his sentence was to pay a fine and submit to regular probationary visits to the local police station. He continued to have an intermittent relationship with his wife and two children. One woman summarized her family dynamics: 'My mother-in-law never thinks her son is the reason for my tragic life incident'. Such experience and sentiment was shared by all study participants.

Perhaps because scarred women are perceived as unfit and as having failed their families, they all reported being excluded from family ceremonies, especially weddings. One woman came to an ear-piercing ceremony (*kadhani vizha*), an important rite of passage for young girls, but was accosted at the door by an angry relative who told the disfigured woman's sister, 'Why did you invite this burned lady?' Embarrassed at having unwittingly created a disturbance, she walked away from the family gathering and did not attend the ceremony.

All women in the two groups had children and most reported severe disruptions in mother–child relationships after they were scarred. All the women in the study groups had been told at least once after their disfigurement that they were now unfit mothers because of their appearance. Several women stated that their relationships with their children were 'normal'; others, however, were denied access to their sons and daughters or said that their appearance frightened their children: 'Even my children will never come to see me', one woman said sadly. Another woman missed her son's wedding, something unheard of in India, for not being wanted because of her appearance. Family members, she said, believed that she was unable and unfit to perform the duties of the mother of the groom and that her presence would undermine the legitimacy of the ceremony.

While their husbands and in-laws deemed all the women inapt or unfit as mothers, two women reported that these relatives also told them that they were unable to become mothers because the kerosene burns made them sterile. 'Everybody said my womb would have been burnt and I will not be able to produce children in the future', one woman said. She went on to say that her husband also made that claim despite knowing that the fire burned her face and hands, not her abdomen. Another woman delivered a healthy baby a year after the disfiguring assault and, as she reported, 'no one believed' that she had given birth.

The participants' families rarely offered a haven from the stigma discrimination encountered in the general public. Although some of the women reported being tolerated at home to various extents, most told of verbal and emotional abuse, neglect, exclusion, and marginalization by parents, siblings, children, and in-laws.

*Threats to Religious Sensibilities:* The second theme indicating the moral menace of disfigurement is that disfigurement threatens certain realities of mainstream Hinduism. India is a country of many religions, but is usually associated with and largely culturally dominated by Hinduism, which was the religion of all but a handful of the women who participated in the study. Four of the participants were Hindu-to-Christian converts, and there were no apparent differences between the victims' stated religion and how they reported others' visions of them. Two related themes were ıost pronounced in the discussions: (1) the Hindu idea of urity and (2) the belief in the magical transformation of umans, especially women, into demons or spirits and the eality of destructive witchcraft, both of which are common omponents in Hindu cosmology.

The Hindu conception of purity is complex and subject to arious meanings and interpretations. Traditional scholars nd religionists envision purity as a sacred concept signifying a ertical continuum of spiritual cleanliness that accounts for a vorldly caste hierarchy and, consequently, the division of abor in India. While some may see purity and pollution in erms of bodily discharges, a belief that classifies women as ess pure than men until women pass through puberty and nenopause, or physical cleanliness, many others say that the urity–pollution continuum runs parallel to a continuum of uspiciousness and inauspiciousness (Klostermaier 2007). Whereas high caste and unpolluted people have a purity of nind and body that comes from good *karma* and the grace of God, lower caste or impure people are placed at the bottom of his order, nearer to demons and sin, for having bad *karma*. Things that 'unclean' people do or touch invoke or portend nauspiciousness, a sign of something bad to come.

As stated earlier, many people refuse to touch objects, particularly tableware, handled by disfigured women, and all he women in the study said they had been turned away from amily gatherings so often that they had given up trying to be nvolved. All of the women in the two groups, however, lenied that these responses were thematically connected to a Hindu sacred concept of purity. Instead, they stated that others treated them *as if* they were polluted or unclean. Although the women agreed that 'they (others) never consider us impure', the behavioral responses of others were not significantly different from those in which sacred impurity is situationally relevant (e.g. caste interaction rules), regardles of the ways they are contextually defined. One woman stated:

> Even if we get into a crowded bus and slightly touch the peopl standing nearby us they will move away and stand. If they move little it means that they are discriminating us and practicin untouchability.

Rather than 'purity as sacred', another religious expla nation may account for the avoidant, untouchability-lik behavior of others. Disfigurement, as all the women agreed was defined by others as a curse (*sapam*) derived from eithe punishment for a past or present life transgression (*karma*) o because the disfigurement transformed the women into super natural beings, or a combination of the two. The disfigure women in the two study groups reported that others ofte believe them to be devils (*saithan*) that hold magical power that are only used to harm or provoke danger. One woma described how this belief manifested in her life:

> My elder brother is an auto driver. His wife considers me to b inauspicious and if my brother sees my face and goes for work, h will have no money gain the whole day, she thinks. She gives a example that if a piece of wood is put in the fire it is a waste an good for nothing. She thinks of me in the same way. And so if I g in front of them she will move away from the path and walk. It i not the strangers, but the family members (who) do such things.

As previously mentioned, disfigured women are rarely, i ever, invited to attend family functions, especially marriage and anything to do with children, for fear they will inten tionally or unintentionally curse the event and the people present. For one victim, the only family events she attended were funerals because there, she said, she could do no magic. The following quotes demonstrate the forms that accusations of demonization take:

> 'They say we look like devils, and so they fear'

'Children scream in fear on seeing me. They will say that the devil is coming'

'People will point me out or recognize me as "burned Mariamman"'[3]

'People say they thought me to be dead, and it's my ghost (*pei*) roaming around. And so they fear seeing me'.

## Conclusion

Little research has been conducted on the sources of particular stigmas. Most of the studies on stigma origins have focused on the origins of stigma sentiments regarding mental illness and disabilities. No research has looked at the basis of facial disfigurement. One study by Marbach and colleagues in 1990 looked at the origins of stigma levied against individuals suffering from chronic facial pain, and this research found that these individuals perceived stigma when their clinician believed that their pain was psychological in nature, rather than physiological, suggesting that the patients had flawed personalities and were the source of their own pain. Such psychologisms are common in social environments that hold individuals responsible for their own psychological wherewithal and deny that social forces have validity in explaining individual behavior. This logic constitutes an example of the classic concept of blaming the victim.

The study presented here similarly contends that the origin of disfigurement stigma is socially constructed. By failing to conform to the standards of religious and social ideals of femininity because of their scarred skin and disfigured features, burned women are held in contempt and believed incapable of performing their expected roles regardless of their actual physical ability. In some cases, stigmatizers seemed to believe that burned women's entire bodies were somehow disabled.

Several years ago, Link, Phelan, and Dovido (2008: 35
developed a typology of the functions of stigma: exploitatio
and domination (keeping people down); norm enforcemer
(keeping people in); and disease avoidance (keeping peop
away). The treatment of burned women fits each dimension c
this hypothesis. Burned women are routinely denied access t
both formal and informal social processes and are punishe
for their appearance and histories. Denying entry to relatior
ships and claiming burned women to be cursed are oppressiv
acts that suppress these women's freedoms to move abou
their communities and even within their family's social spac
By using social standards of women's expectations in famil
life and religious sentiments to control burned women's soci
actions, society is reinforcing the expectations of women i
general as well as legitimating the act of burning. The absenc
of active police and judicial enforcement of the law support
not so tacitly that women who do not fit the ideal ar
expendable. Finally, the stigma against burned wome
provides means to avoidance. To not associate with burne
women, as the burned women in the focus groups clearl
stated is a routine response to their appearance, means not t
taint one's own social standing.

Women who survive burn attacks display the fact tha
they were burned every minute of every day. They canno
deny or hide their history. Nor can they conceal the scars as
sign to others that they are damaged physically. Unfortunatel
the scars signal to others that something is wrong with them a
human beings, that their very humanness is tainted, spoiled
and somehow dangerous. They are clearly feared, not becaus
of their behavior or character, but because of the meanings o
their appearance in the context of the expectations o
womanhood in an ages-old and well-entrenched patriarchy
Burned women, in the patriarch's mind, are not attractiv
physically or culturally, and therefore not desirable and ar

denied the opportunity to engage in normative society and relationships.

As the *Manusmriti* (5/158) states:

> Women have no divine right to perform any religious ritual, nor make vows or observe a fast. Her only duty is to obey and please her husband and she will for that reason alone be exalted in heaven.

When women are burned, they are denied even the barest of traditional religious and familial expectations, and thus refused divine exaltation. Women's value is quickly cheapened when they are scarred, which shows the low value they had before the assault. To become so demeaned simply because of their appearance indicates how fragile women's position is in everyday life. Therefore, we can say that to burn is to kill, even if the body survives.

## Notes

1. Portions of this chapter were previously published as Furr, L. Allen. 2014. Facial disfigurement stigma: A study of victims of domestic assaults with fire in India. *Violence Against Women*, 20(7): 783–798.
2. My university's Institutional Review Board and the ethics review panel of the supporting agency approved the study's research design and protocol.
3. Mariamman is the primary goddess figure in southern India, especially Tamil Nadu where the study was conducted. Mariamman is associated with rain and fertility and is the protector against contagious diseases such as small pox and measles. A 'burned' Mariamman would constitute an ominous sign with prophetic significance.

# 5
# Conclusions

> 'The most common way people give up their power is by thinking they don't have any'.
>
> —Alice Walker

This study has attempted to make sociological sense of the stories of Indian women who have been attacked with fire by their husbands. The data show that after women are attacked by kerosene fire they experience two more traumas in their lives. First, 'society' changes their identities from whom they were before the attack to a new identity that includes being disfigured. They are no longer 'a woman'; they are transformed into 'a burned woman'. Second, because that identity change is dramatic and permanent, disfigured women to varying degrees are socially excommunicated. This migration in status and identity exemplifies Goffman's (1961) concept of the degradation ceremony where disfigured women, who despite good health and functionality, are interpreted by others as having little worth or appeal because their appearance is marred by scars. Their disfigured appearance, in dramaturgical language, becomes their master status, which can be defined as a quality or status position that dominates all others held by the person. A master status is centrally defining; it is the characteristic that constitutes the nebulas of a person's social identity.

Using Yang et al.'s (2007) analysis as a theoretical guide, the analysis of the data in this study yielded two themes that shed light on explaining the stigma these women reported. First, disfigurement stigma is related to threats to normative family life. The fitness of disfigured women to fulfill roles of wife and mother were routinely questioned and demeaned. A second theme, disfigurement as threatening to religious sensibilities, suggests that women burned by fire were believed transformed into supernatural beings capable of ruining daily life processes and rituals by applying magical curses. The themes extracted from these data lend support to Yang et al.'s theory that stigma occurs in the ebb and flow of daily life and is attached to those qualities that endanger the norms and values of everyday existence. The question arises, therefore, as to what sociocultural system regulates everyday life and triggers the negative evaluation of a disfigured face.

Disfigurement stigma in India occurs in the social context of the Indian patriarchy where women, as a general rule, are dependent upon men for social status and identity and economic well-being. As Nussbaum (2000: 220) states, women in India are not necessarily treated as 'ends in their own rights'; that is, as persons with opportunities to choose and pursue life goals from an array of choices beyond the traditional roles of wife and mother. Rather, women are valued and defined by their instrumental worth as vehicles intended to promote the ends of male achievement and fulfillment (Nussbaum 2000). Women's life chances, consequently, are typically limited to that of caregivers, sexual outlets, son producers, and laborers. Disfigurement stigma further removes burned women from those already limited roles.

This objectification of women's instrumentality implies that women should possess the native characteristics necessary to be successful in such a system. These qualities, which include obedience, chastity, and physical beauty, are taught to most Indian girls as models set forth by the exemplars of the feminine persona. Girls and women are expected to follow the ideal life paths of Sita and Savitri, among others, who, in Hindu lore, represent female humbleness and allegiance to men (Hess 1999; Mukherjee 1999). In particular, Sita's purity, obedience, and sacrifice in the service of men symbolize the national representation of ideal womanhood (Bhattacharya 2000; Zacharias 2001). These characteristics are commonly instilled in young girls as the embodiment of self-realization and personal fulfillment. For Sita's dedication to be meaningful and perhaps even relevant, however, she first had to be beautiful.

As further indication of disfigurement as a master status, social psychological research confirms that people within and across cultures judge and treat others based on attractiveness (Langlois et al. 2000). In India, these reactions include gendered variations that often have substantial and significant consequences. Feminist accounts of the value placed on female attractiveness pose strong arguments for a dual system of perception when comparing and assessing male and female appearance. Attractiveness clearly holds more social capital value for girls and women than for boys and men (Bhattacharya 2000; Dutta 2003). Female facial appearance, for example, is a primary bargaining card in arranging marriages, which remain the norm in India. More attractive women can move up in caste rank via a well negotiated marital arrangement, which improves not only the daughter's economic well-being, but that of her family of origin as well.

In a culture where the pressure to 'marry off' daughters has social and economic implications, parents fret over the tone of their daughters' skin, the shape of their teeth, and whether or not they will require spectacles to improve their vision, often spending money they can ill afford in order to correct perceived flaws and improve their daughters' attractiveness to men (Oldenburg 2002). 'Plain' daughters are a liability: the longer they remain unmarried, the longer parents must support them. Further, less attractive daughters are a source of shame and incur higher dowry costs to improve their appeal to potential husbands (Oldenburg 2002). None of the extensive literature on Indian mate selection and gender relationships describes a comparable emphasis on male appearance.

A similar reasoning applies in disfigurement stigma. In a patriarchal world, adult women thought to be unattractive have little sexual value and in time become economic and emotional burdens. Since the sexual worth of disfigured women has been destroyed, so has their very personhood. The stigma turns these women into soiled beings and repels sympathy that ought to go to them as victims of domestic violence and attempted homicide.

Demonizing women has a long history in Indian religious thinking and folklore, and disfigured women in particular have symbolized evil and sin (Wilson 1996). From hagiographies and current interpretations of the disfigured female body, we see the continuity of the belief that a mutilated face is perceived as a fitting punishment for a woman who, as Wilson relates, has revealed her true inner nature. Such a woman is marked as supernatural, malevolent, and wicked; one that should be avoided at all costs.

In sum, the forms that stigma take may represent disfigured women's failure to maintain the norms and values that govern the expectations of womanhood. Disfigurement, as suggested by the stigma, violates wide-reaching core values that define the ideals of Indian femininity, which hold that women's highest achievements are as wife and mother and maintaining beauty and sexual allure. If women lose their attractiveness, they are unfit to be a part of a marriage, which by definition in the Indian social context means they cannot preserve the core family structure. Consequently when women are judged as unable to perpetuate the family, they are demonized, feared, and religiously sanctioned.

Disfigurement stigma is a product of presumed threats to the moral order of everyday life that disfigurement is presumed to pose. This moral order, which is rooted in the extensive web of South Asian patriarchal norms, values, and social organization, specifies particularistic expectations of women's appearance, and if these expectations are violated via disfigurement, stigma and social exclusion follow.

Stigma, therefore, should be considered a sumptuary rule in a society. Sumptuary rules are morality-based standards that enforce social rankings and hierarchies. Originally such norms were codified into law and were designed to regulate consumption of certain foods, items of clothing, furniture, and other articles that could be considered indicators of social standing. The idea was to restrict access to certain commodities to elites to make it easy to identify social rank and privilege (Ribeiro 2003). Sumptuary rules are important for social classification systems and have evolved to include more than access to or possession of certain things. Nowadays sumptuary norms stratify people based on their perceived moral standing.

As Karen Fields and Barbara Fields wrote in their interesting book *Racecraft*, 'they (sumptuary rules) do what nature leaves undone' (2012: 33). Nature does not cause human social variations. There are no sub-species or breeds of humans. Stratification of humans into groups of rich and poor or good and bad is a product of social activities. Nonetheless, there are many who want nature to explain human differences. Their reasoning is that if there are natural variations in the human animal, then mistreatment or the denial of 'the good things in life' is justifiable. Just as we do not give civil rights to horses, fish, and snakes, so should we not provide for 'lesser humans', according to this way of thinking.

Sumptuary rules provide a pseudo-scientific and subjective explanation for justifying and reinforcing social hierarchies in the absence of natural explanations of what appears to be natural differences in people. As a type of such norms, disfigurement stigma forces an 'us' and 'other' social classification onto people based on an interpretation of physical (and therefore 'natural') attributes and characteristics. Disfigurement 'seems' to be a fact of nature – the body is changed and presumed less than normal with its scars and deformities. The rules of stigma therefore seem legitimate by defining a scheme rooted in the apparent inferiority and superiority of disfigured and non-disfigured people, respectively. These rules are enforced by nativistic rituals such as denying disfigured women certain religious ceremonies and banning them from social affairs and aspects of everyday life such as taking meals together. Because sumptuary norms are presumed to explain natural human divisions, they are followed mechanically as if they were ordained by a natural order of the universe. Furthermore, the seemingly naturalness of stigma makes it practically impossible for the people who hold these beliefs to understand stigma as a subjective social creation (Fields and Fields 2012). The forest is hidden behind the trees.

I consider stigma as an emotional reaction within an ideology of oppression. Relatedly, the Fields sisters, in talking about race in the United States, stated that people are perceived as naturally inferior when they are already seen as a conquered group. In other words, stigma is a self-evident, inevitable natural law applied to a group that falls under the control of another. The oppressed group, in this view, is innately inferior and essentialized by virtue of being dominated. Consequently ideology develops to 'prove' that inferiority of which stigma is part. Stigma plays a role in this web of power by denying the humanness of women. Men who subscribe to this line of thinking successfully classify girls and women as an 'other', a 'not us' group of people within their own communities and families. Extraordinary as this appears, controlling women's sexuality and basic freedoms has benefits for men, not the least of which is providing them with a sense of social command. By denigrating sexual differences, men exert control and require obedience, allowing them to hold social power and prestige.

Disfigurement stigma is an excellent illustration of these mechanisms. Disfigured women are treated as pariah because women are already oppressed: they are easy targets for the patriarchy. The stigma levied against disfigured women is gendered; there are sexual connotations to it that do not appear in how disfigured men are treated. Being cast as demons or thought to be unable to perform the social roles assigned to women, even when they are able, tells us that disfigured women are failed beings, unable to perform the duties assigned to them as oppressed persons. They are a threat to the establishment of a moral order that requires female attractiveness and instrumentality that serve the needs of fathers, husbands, and sons. Men, paradoxically, create the threat themselves: they first construct patriarchal social rules, attack women violently, and then stigmatize survivors.

There is an old and simplistic adage for explaining domestic and intimate violence against women: Men hit women because they can. The idea is that men initiate and perpetuate violence because there are few barriers prohibiting them. Men, on average, are stronger and more powerful physically than women; yet what accounts for the persistence of domestic violence is not sheer brawn, but the social controls that are too weak to prevent their violent behavior. Law enforcement cites domestic violence as a 'low status' crime.

Women find little recourse in the courts. But more importantly, moral social constraints provide relatively little influence. Many men, about one-third of Indian men in fact,[1] believe they have the right to hit, punch, or burn the women whom they feel entitled to master. The patriarchy allows them permission to control women with any means possible. If essentialism suggests that women are interchangeable, burning them indicates their disposability. Not only are women one-dimensional and essentially the same person, the single female personage is characterized as impure and potentially dangerous, requiring cleansing and discarding if necessary.

The disfigured female body has been discredited through the discourse of patriarchy and the mechanism of stigma. The biological body, therefore, no longer exists. It has been reconstituted as and replaced by a socially constructed invention – the disfigured woman. This new construction is an intersection of two statuses, being female and disfigured, which subjects these women to new denigrations and new restraints above and beyond the marginalization they encounter as ordinary women.

Internalized as an object that is envisioned as dangerous and all bad, the image of the disfigured woman in India has become a mythologized motif. The disfigured female face is given a hostile and dangerous meaning against which stigmatizers feel impelled to defend themselves. The disfigured face of an 'other' is threatening to both oneself and one's community, and therefore must be rebuked.

## Hope

From my meetings with disfigured Indian women, I have learned of the great resiliency and determination of women who struggle not only against the daily stresses and hassles of everyday life, but also against the unjust demands and marginalization of a broad social system that is rigged against them. Apart from the sociological insights gleaned from the analytical parts of the analysis, the study influenced my own growth as a person and as a member of the global community. India is not my culture or nation; India, however, is my teacher. Each time I travel to the subcontinent, I return to my own home with fresh insights into the human condition not just about India, but also of all humankind.

On this particular trip, I learned firsthand of the ability of people to act sadistically. I saw the inhumanity and the emotional and physical consequences of hatred, ignorance, and selfishness. To lay eyes upon the horrific scars on women's skin, hands with missing fingers, and the countless other impairments caused by someone whom they promised to nurture and support but who intentionally burn them alive is not and should not be a value-neutral, objective or purely scientific experience.

I've climbed the steps to meet Gita many times in my mind since that hot summer day, and I cannot shake the emotions that were evoked seeing her lying on that cot, wounded and abased, and hearing her story. Rarely have I felt such sorrow.

Despite my encounter with such misery, I also learned of the champion nature of the human spirit and of how to overcome injustice and avoid misery. The stories of women in this study were not completely despairing or hopeless. Consistent with Western studies that report that many severely disfigured persons adjust to the social and psychological demands forced onto them because of their appearance (see Robinson's 1997 review), the majority of the women in the focus groups reported upon here, in varying degrees, have learned to cope with their appearance and the accompanying stigma. They have accepted the loss of their appearance and the roles they held before they were burned, and they have offset the losses with a renewed vigor about their lives as women and as mothers. Many displayed a delightful sense of humor and were working to re-invent themselves as women in control of their lives.

The most lasting image I have retained from this study is that of women asserting their own agency, rejecting the principles of patriarchal expectations, and carving out a place for themselves by making sense of their circumstances through proactive decision-making and contesting assertions that contradict their own self-assessment. Two participants in the study were particularly inspiring. Both were living as heads of their households and without their husbands, and vividly described their feelings of empowerment and the progression of their own social autonomy. Confidence, emotional strength, and fortitude enabled them to support themselves and their children without aid from their husbands or other family members or charity. These women were self-employed and had jobs that generated an income sufficient to provide food, housing, and a penance of discretionary spending. Furthermore, they felt adequately comfortable with their appearance that they would argue with people who made disparaging comments to them. Taking pride in their accomplishments, both women couched their resiliency in feminist terms. As one said, 'Women, including me, are developing vastly in all fields. Women no longer need men'.

## Notes

1. Virtually every study investigating the incidence and prevalence of domestic and intimate partner violence in India reports that about one-third of ever-married women have experienced violence at the hands of their husbands. The DHS men's panel asks men if beating their wives is justified under various situations. Over 37 per cent said yes, if his wife shows disrespect to her in-laws, and about 31 per cent agreed that beatings are justified if his wife neglects their children. Just under 26 per cent of men said that wife beating is justified if his wife argues with him.

# Bibliography


Agarwal, Bina. 1998. Widows versus daughters or widows as daughters? Property, land, and economic security in rural India. *Modern Asian Studies*, 32(1): 1–48.

Alexander, Caroline. 2007. Faces of war. *The Smithsonian*. Retrieved from http://www.smithsonianmag.com/history/faces-of-war–145799854/?no-ist=&=&page=1. Accessed on 12 April 2016.

Basu, S. 1999. *She Comes to Take Her Rights*. Albany: State University of New York Press.

Batra, A.K. 2003. Burn mortality: Recent trends and sociocultural determinants in rural India. *Burns*, 29(3): 270–5.

Belur, Jyoti, Nick Tilley, Nayreen Daruwall, Meena Kumar, Vinay Tiwari, and Dagid Osrin. 2014. The social construction of 'dowry deaths'. *Social Science and Medicine*, 119: 1–9.

Berreman, Gerald D. 1992. Sanskritization of female oppression in India. In *Sex and Gender Hierarchies*, Barbara Diane Miller (ed.), pp. 366–92. Cambridge: Cambridge University Press.

Bhargava, Anju P. 2000. Contemporary influence of Sita. Retrieved from http://www.infinityfoundation.com/mandala/s_es/s_es_bharg_sita_frameset.htm. Accessed on 5 December 2016.

Bhattacharya, M. 2000. Iron bangles to iron shackles: A study of women's marriage and subordination within poor households in Calcutta. *Man in India*, 80(1–2): 1–29.

Biddle J. E. and D. S. Hamermesh. 1998. Beauty, productivity, and discrimination: Lawyers' looks and lucre. *Journal of Labor Economics*, 16(1): 172–201.

Bloch, F., V. Rao, and S. Desai. 2004. Wedding celebrations as conspicuous consumption: Signalling social status in rural India. *Journal of Human Resources*, 39(3): 675–95.

Bourdieu, Pierre. 1977. *Outline of a Theory of Practice*. Cambridge and New York: Cambridge University Press.

Bourdieu, Pierre and L.J.D. Wacquant. 1992. *An Invitation to Reflexive Sociology*. Chicago and London: University of Chicago Press.

Brown, George William. 1921/2016. *The Human Body in the Upanishads*. Delhi, India: Facsimile Publisher.

Bull, Ray and Julia Stevens. 1981. The effects of facial disfigurement on helping behaviour. *Italian Journal of Psychology*, 8(1): 25–33.

CNN. 2003. Indian woman and baby burned alive for dowry, policy say. Retrieved from http://myfox8.com/2014/02/03/indian-woman-and-baby-burned-alive-for-dowry-police-say/. Accessed on 22 January 2017.

Compton, Herbert. 1904. *Indian Life in Town and Country*. New York: G.P. Putnam's Sons.

Currie, Thomas E. and Anthony C. Little. 2009. The relative importance of the face and body in judgments of human physical attractiveness. *Evolution and Human Behavior*, 30: 409–16.

Das Gupta, M. 1987. Selective discrimination against female children in rural Punjab, India. *Population and Development Review*, 13(1): 77–100.

Datta, V.N. 1988. *Sati: A Historical, Social, and Philosophical Enquiry into the Hindu Rite of Widow Burning*. Riverdale, MD: Riverdale Co.

de Beauvoir, Simone. 1973. *The Second Sex*. New York: Vintage Books.

Demographic and Health Surveys (India) (Iair52sv). 2006a. USAID, Calverton, MD.

Demographic and Health Surveys (India) (Iamr52fl). 2006b. USAID, Calverton, MD.

Dutta, R.K. 2003. *Crime Against Women*. New Delhi: Reference Press.

Ellsberg M., H.A. Jansen, L. Heise, C.H. Watts, C. and Garcia-Moreno. 2008. Intimate partner violence and women's physical and mental health in the WHO multi-country study on women's health and domestic violence: An observational study. *Lancet*, 371: 1165–72.

England, Paula. 2016. Sometimes the social becomes personal: Gender, class, and sexualities. *American Sociological Review*, 81(1): 4–28.

Falk, Gerhard. 2001. *Stigma: How We Treat Outsiders*. Amherst, NY: Prometheus Books.

Fields, Karen E. and Barbara J. Fields. 2012. *Racecraft: The Soul of Inequality in American Life*. New York: Verso.

Furr, L. Allen. 1997. *Exploring Human Behavior and the Social Environment*. Boston: Allyn and Bacon.

Furr, L. Allen. 2014. Facial disfigurement stigma: A study of victims of domestic assaults with fire in India. *Violence Against Women*, 20(7): 783–98.

Furr, L. Allen, Osborne Wiggins, Michael Cunningham, Dalibor Vasilic, Charles S. Brown, Joseph C. Banis, Claudio Maldonado, Gustavo Perez-Abadia, and John H. Barker. 2007. Psychosocial implications of disfigurement and the future of human face transplantation. *Plastic and Reconstructive Surgery*, 120(2): 559–65.

Garcia-Moreno, Claudio. 2009. Gender inequality and fire-related deaths in India. *Lancet*, 373: 1230–1231.

Gecas, Viktor. 1989. The social psychology of self-efficacy. *Annual Review of Sociology*, 15: 291–316.

Gehrsitz, Markus. 2014. Looks and labor: Do attractive people work more? *Lancet*, 28(3): 269–87.

George, Abraham. 2005. *India Untouched: The Forgotten Face of Rural Poverty*. Cranston, RI (USA): The Writers' Collective.

Goffman, Erving. 1961. *Asylums: Essays on the Social Situation of Mental Patients and other Inmates*. New York: Anchor Books.

Goffman, Erving. 1963. *Stigma: Notes on the Management of Spoiled Identity*. Englewood Cliffs, NJ: Prentice-Hall.

Grealy, Lucy. 1994. *Autobiography of a Face*. Boston: Houghton Mifflin.

Hamby, Sherry and John Grych. 2013. *The Web of Violence: Exploring Connections among Different Forms of Interpersonal Violence and Abuse*. New York: Springer.

Hamermesh, Daniel. S. and Jeff E. Biddle. 1994. Beauty and the labor market. *The American Economic Review*, 84(5): 1174–94.

Harlan, Lindsey. 1994. Perfection and devotion: Sati tradition in Rajasthan. In *Sati, The Blessing and the Curse: The Burning of Wives in India*, John Stratton Hawley (ed.), pp. 79–99. New York: Oxford University Press.

Harper, B. 2000. Beauty, stature and the labor market: A British cohort study. *Oxford Bulletin of Economics and Statistics*, 62(Special issue): 771–800.

Hess, Linda. 1999. Rejecting Sita: Indian responses to the ideal man's cruel treatment of his ideal wife. *Journal of the American Academy of Religion*, 67(1): 1–32.

Hochschild, Arlie Russell. 1983. *The Managed Heart: Commercialization of Human Feeling*. Berkeley: University of California Press.

Houska, William. 1981. The characteristics of son preference in an urban scheduled caste community. *The Eastern Anthropologist*, 34: 1.

Houston, Vicky and Ray Bull. 1994. Do people avoid sitting next to someone who is facially disfigured? *European Journal of Social Psychology*, 24(2): 279–84.

*India's Daughter: The Life of Jyoti Singh*. 2012. Leslee Udwin, Director and Producer.

Jaiswal, Ashish K., Himanshu Aggarwal, Pooja Solanki, P.S. Lubana, R.K. Mathur, and Sudarshan Odiya. 2007. Epidemiological and socio-cultural study of burn patients in M.Y. Hospital, Indore, India. *Indian Journal of Plastic Surgery*, 40(2): 158–63.

Jejeebhoy, S.J. and R. Cook. 1997. State accountability for wife beating: The Indian challenge. *Lancet, Women's Health Supplement*, 33: 855–62.

Judge, Timothy A., Charlice Hurst, and Lauren S. Simon. 2009. Does it pay to be smart, attractive, or confident (or all three)? Relationships among general mental ability, physical attractiveness, core self-evaluations, and income. *Journal of Applied Psychology*, 94(3): 742–55.

Kishwar, Madhu. 1994. Codified Hindu law: Myth and reality. *Economic and Political Weekly*, 29: 2145–161.

Klostermaier, Klaus K. 2007. *A Survey of Hinduism*, 3rd edition. Albany: State University of New York Press.

Kohn, Melvin L. and Carmi Schooler. 1973. Occupational experience and psychological functioning: An assessment of reciprocal effects. *American Sociological Review*, 38(1): 97–118.

Kroska, Amy and Sarah K. Harkness. 2006. Stigma sentiments and self-meanings: Exploring the modified labeling theory of mental illness. *Social Psychology Quarterly*, 69(4): 325–48.

Kumar, S.C., S.D. Gupta, and G. Abraham. 2002. Masculinity and violence against women in marriage: An exploratory study in Rajasthan. In *Men, Masculinity and Domestic Violence in India: Summary Report of Four Studies*, International Centre for Research on Women (ed.). Washington, DC: International Centre for Research on Women. Retrieved from https://www.icrw.org/wp-content/uploads/2016/10/Domestic-Violence-in-India–4-Men-Masculinity-and-Domestic-Violence-in-India.pdf. Accessed on 15 June 2017.

Kumar, Sanchil, Uma Shankar Singh, Anoop K. Verma, Wahid Ali, and Akhilesh Krishna. 2014. Intentional and non-intentional burn related deaths: A comparative study of socio-demographic profile. *Burns*. doi: 10.1016/j.burns.2014.06.006.

Kumar, Sanchil, Wahid Ali, Anoop K. Verma, Abhishek Pandey, and Shiuli Rathore. 2013. Epidemiology and mortality of burns in the Lucknow region, India: A 5-Year study. *Burns*, 39(8): 1599–605.

Kumar, Virendra. 2003. Burnt wives: A study of suicides. *Burns*, 29: 31–5.

Kumar, Virendra and C.B. Tripathi. 2004. Burnt wives: A study of homicides. *Medical Science and Law*, 44(1): 55–60.

Lal, Ruby. 2013. *Coming of Age in Nineteenth-Century India: The Girl-Child and the Art of Playfulness.* Cambridge, UK: Cambridge University Press.

Langlois, J.H., L. Kalakanis, A.J. Rubenstein, A. Larson, M. Hallam, and M. Smoot. 2000. Maxims or myths of beauty? A meta-analytic and theoretical review. *Psychological Bulletin*, 126: 390–423.

Levine, Elie, Linda Degutis, Thomas Pruzinsky, Joseph Shin, and John A. Persing. 2005. Quality of life and facial trauma: Psychological and body image effects. *Annals of Plastic Surgery*, 54(5): 502–10.

Link, Bruce G. 1987. Understanding labeling effects in the area of mental disorders: An assessment of the effects of expectations of rejection. *American Sociological Review*, 52: 96–112.

Link, Bruce G. and Jo C. Phelan. 2001. Conceptualizing stigma. *Annual Review of Sociology*, 27: 363–85.

Link, Bruce G., Jo C. Phelan, and John F. Dovido. 2008. Stigma and prejudice: One animal or two? *Social Science and Medicine*, 67(3): 358–67.

Macgregor, Francis Cooke. 1951. Some psycho-social problems associated with facial deformities. *American Sociological Review*, 16(5): 629–38.

Macgregor, Francis Cooke. 1990. Facial disfigurement: Problems and management of social interaction and implications for mental health. *Aesthetic Plastic Surgery*, 14: 249–57.

Marbach, Joseph J., Mary Clare Lennon, Bruce G. Link, and Bruce P. Dohrenwend. 1990. Losing face: Sources of stigma as perceived by chronic facial pain patients. *Journal of Behavioral Medicine*, 13(6): 583–604.

Mehta, Kalyani K. 2011. The challenges of conducting focus-group research among Asian older adults. *Ageing and Society*, 31(3): 408–21.

Ministry of Home Affairs. 2010. National Crime Records Bureau. *Accidental Deaths and Suicide in India 2010*. New Delhi, India.

Ministry of Home Affairs. 2013. National Crime Records Bureau. *Crime in India 2013*. New Delhi, India.

Mobius, M.M. and T.S. Rosenblat. 2006. Why beauty matters. *The American Economic Review*, 96(1): 222–35.

Morgan, David L. 1996. Focus groups. *Annual Review of Sociology*, 22: 129–52.

Mukherjee, Prabhati. 1999. *Hindu Women: Normative Models*. Hyderabad: Orient Longman.

Narayan, Uma. 1997. Cross-cultural connections, border-crossings, and 'death by culture'. In *Dislocating Cultures/Identities, Traditions, and*

*Third-World Feminism*, Uma Narayan (ed.), pp. 83–117. New York: Routledge Press.

Nussbaum, Martha. 2000. Women's capabilities and social justice. *Journal of Human Development*, 1: 219–47.

Oldenburg, Veena Talwar. 2002. *Dowry Murder: The Imperial Origins of a Cultural Crime*. Oxford: Oxford University Press.

Olivelle, Patrick. 2005. *Manu's Code of Law*. Oxford: Oxford University Press.

Padubidri, J.R., R.G. Meneges, S. Pant, and S.B. Shetty. 2013. Deaths among women of reproductive age: A forensic autopsy study. *Journal of Forensic and Legal Medicine*, 20(6): 651–4.

Pande, Rohini and Nan Marie Astone. 2007. Explaining son preference in rural India: The independent role of structural versus individual factors. *Population Research and Policy Review,* 26(1).

Parker, Richard, and Peter Aggleton. 2003. HIV and AIDS-related stigma and discrimination: A conceptual framework and implications for action. *Social Science and Medicine*, 57: 13–24.

Parr, Lisa A. 2011. The evolution of face processing in primates. *Philosophical Transactions of the Royal Society*, 366: 1764–77.

Patel, Vikam, Chinthanie Ramasundarahettige, Lakshmi Vijaykumar, J.S. Thakur, Vendhan Gajalakshmi, Gopalkrishna Gururaj, Wilson Suraweera, and Prabhat Jha. 2012. Suicide mortality in India: A nationally representative survey. *Lancet*, 379(9834): 23–9.

Peck, M.D. 2012. Epidemiology of burns throughout the world. Part II: Intentional burns in adults. *Burns*, 38(5): 630–7.

Prentice, D.A. and D.T. Miller. 2006. Essentializing differences between women and men. *Psychological Science*, 17(2): 129–35. doi: 10.1111/j.1467-9280.2006.01675.x.

Pruzinsky, Thomas. 1992. Social and psychological effects of major craniofacial deformity. *The Cleft Palate-Craniofacial Journal*, 29(6): 578–84.

Pruzinsky, Thomas, Elie Levine, John A. Persing, Jeffrey T. Barth, and Robert Obrecht. 2005. Facial trauma and facial cancer. In *Psychological Aspects of Reconstructive and Cosmetic Plastic Surgery*, Sawyer, David B., Pruzinsky, Thomas, Cash, Thomas F., Goldwyn, Robert M., Persing, John A., and Whitaker, Linton A (eds), pp. 125–144. Philadelphia: Lippincott Williams and Wilkins.

Qayyam, Kanal. Quoted in 'Losing soul after face hurts more, says acid attack victim', by Hason Mansoor on Dawn.com 1 February 2014. Accessed on 23 July 2014.

Renz, Evan M. and Leopoldo C. Cancio. 2012. Acute Burn Care. Retrieved from http://www.cs.amedd.army.mil/borden/book/ccc/UCLAchp12.pdf. Accessed on 15 June 2017.<Publisher: Please check the URL. I am not able to check the URL.>

Ribeiro, Aileen. 2003. *Dress and Morality*. London: Berg Publishers.

Robinson, E. 1997. *Psychological Research on Visible Difference in Adults*. London: Butterworth Heinemann.

Robitaille, Marie-Claire. 2013. Determinants of stated son preference in India: Are men and women different? *The Journal of Development Studies*, 49(5): 657–69.

Rudd, Jane. 2001. Dowry-murder: An example of violence against women. *Women's International Forum*, 24(5): 513–22.

Rumsey, Nichola, Ray Bull, and Denis Gahanna. 1982. The effect of facial disfigurement on the proxemic behavior of the general public. *Journal of Applied Social Psychology*, 12(2): 137–50.

Rumsey, Nichola, Alex Clarke, Paul White, Menna Wyn-Williams, and Wendy Garlick. 2004. Altered body image: Appearance-related concerns of people with visible disfigurement. *Journal of Advanced Nursing*, 48(5): 443–53

Sanghavi, P., K. Bhalla, and V. Das. 2009. Fire-related deaths in India in 2001: A retrospective analysis of data. *Lancet*, 373(96712): 1282–8.

Sawhney, C. 1989. Flame burns involving kerosene pressure stoves in India. *Burns*, 15(6): 362–4.

Sen, Mala. 2001. *Sati, Dowry Death, and Female Infanticide in Modern India*. New Brunswick, NJ: Rutgers University Press.

Shaha, K. and S. Mohanty. 2006. Alleged dowry death: A study of homicidal burns. *Medical Science and Law*, 46(2): 105–10.

Shahidul B. M. and C. I. Mahmud. 2001. Acid burns in Bangladesh. *Annals of Burns Disasters*, 14: 115–18.

Shahidul, B.M., M. Choudhary, and I. Mahmud. 2001. Acid burns in Bangladesh. *Annals of Burns and Fire Disorders*, XIV(3).

Sharma, B., D. Harish, V. Sharma, and K. Vij. 2002. Kitchen accidents vis-à-vis dowry deaths. *Burns*, 28(3): 250–3.

Shilling, Chris. 2005. *The Body in Culture, Technology and Society*. London: Sage Publications.

Simmel, George. 1964. *The Sociology of Georg Simmel*, Kurt H. Wolff (translator). New York: Free Press.

Srinivasan, Padma and Gary R. Lee. 2004. The dowry system in northern India: Women's attitudes and social change. *Journal of Marriage and Family*, 66: 1108–17.

Srivastava, Amitabh. 2016. Over 2000 women killed in India for practicing 'black magic' in 14 years. *India Today*. Retrieved from http://indiatoday.intoday.in/story/over–2000-women-killed-in-india-for-practicing-black-magic-in–14-years/1/696147.html. Accessed on 12 December 2016.

Stevenage, Sarah V. and Yolanda McKay. 1999. Model applicant: The effect of facial appearance on recruitment decisions. *British Journal of Psychology*, 90(2): 221–34.

Stone, Alison. 2007. *An Introduction to Feminist Philosophy*. Cambridge, UK: Polity Press.

Stone, Linda and Carolyn James. 1995. Dowry, bride-burning, and female power in India. *Women's Studies International Forum*, 18(2): 125–34.

Synnott, Anthony. 1989. Truth and goodness, mirrors and masks – part I: A sociology of beauty and the face. *British Journal of Sociology*, 40(4): 607–36.

*Times of India*. 2009. Why Sati is still a burning issue. Retrieved from http://timesofindia.indiatimes.com/Why-sati-is-still-a-burning-issue/articleshow/4897797.cms. Accessed on 24 April 2016.

*Times of India*. 2013. Dowry deaths: One woman dies every hour. Retrieved from http://timesofindia.indiatimes.com/india/Dowry-deaths-One-woman-dies-every-hour/articleshow/22201659.cms. Accessed on 21 July 2016.

Trachtenberg, Alan. 2000. Lincoln's smile: Ambiguities of the face in photography. *Social Research*, 67(1): 1–25.

Umar, Mohd. 1998. *Bride Burning in India: A Socio Legal Study*. New Delhi: A.P.H. Publishing Corporation.

Wacquant, Loic. 2005. *Pierre Bourdieu and Democratic Politics: The Mystery of Ministry*. Malden, MA: Polity Press.

Walker, Lenore E. 1979. *The Battered Woman*. New York: Harper and Row.

Walters, E. 1997. *Psychological Research on Visible Difference in Adults*. London: Butterworth Heinemann.

Wilson, Liz. 1996. *Charming Cadavers: Horrific Figurations of the Feminine in Indian Buddhist Hagiographic Literature*. Chicago: University of Chicago Press.

Witt, Charlotte. 2011. *The Metaphysics of Gender*. New York: Oxford University Press.

World Health Organization. 2009. *Suicide Prevention*, 2009. Geneva: World Health Organization.

World Health Organization. 2016. *Burns*. Geneva: World Health Organization.

Yang, Lawrence Hsin, Arthur Kleinman, Bruce Link, Jo C. Phelan, Sing Lee, Byron Good. 2007. Culture and stigma: Adding moral experience to stigma theory. *Social Science and Medicine*, 64: 1524–35.

Zacharias, Usha. 2001. Trial by fire: Gender, power, and citizenship in narratives of the nation. *Social Text*, 19(4): 29–51.

# Index